NATIONAL INSTITUTES OF HEALTH TOOLBOX COGNITION BATTERY (NIH TOOLBOX CB): VALIDATION FOR CHILDREN BETWEEN 3 AND 15 YEARS

EDITED BY

Philip David Zelazo

Patricia J. Bauer

WITH COMMENTARY BY

Nathan A. Fox

Patricia J. Bauer
Series Editor*

MONOGRAPHS OF THE SOCIETY FOR RESEARCH IN CHILD DEVELOPMENT

Serial No. 309, Vol. 78, No. 4, 2013

*This monograph was accepted under the editorship of W. Andrew Collins.

WILEY Boston, Massachusetts   Oxford, United Kingdom

EDITOR
PATRICIA J. BAUER
Emory University

MANAGING EDITOR
ADAM MARTIN
Society for Research in Child Development

EDITORIAL ASSISTANT
STEPHANIE DEFOUW
Society for Research in Child Development

NATIONAL INSTITUTES OF HEALTH TOOLBOX COGNITION BATTERY (NIH TOOLBOX CB): VALIDATION FOR CHILDREN BETWEEN 3 AND 15 YEARS

CONTENTS

I. NIH TOOLBOX COGNITION BATTERY (CB): INTRODUCTION AND PEDIATRIC DATA
Sandra Weintraub, Patricia J. Bauer, Philip David Zelazo, Kathleen Wallner-Allen, Sureyya S. Dikmen, Robert K. Heaton, David S. Tulsky, Jerry Slotkin, David L. Blitz, Noelle E. Carlozzi, Richard J. Havlik, Jennifer L. Beaumont, Dan Mungas, Jennifer J. Manly, Beth G. Borosh, Cindy J. Nowinski, and Richard C. Gershon 1

II. NIH TOOLBOX COGNITION BATTERY (CB): MEASURING EXECUTIVE FUNCTION AND ATTENTION
Philip David Zelazo, Jacob E. Anderson, Jennifer Richler, Kathleen Wallner-Allen, Jennifer L. Beaumont, and Sandra Weintraub 16

III. NIH TOOLBOX COGNITION BATTERY (CB): MEASURING EPISODIC MEMORY
Patricia J. Bauer, Sureyya S. Dikmen, Robert K. Heaton, Dan Mungas, Jerry Slotkin, and Jennifer L. Beaumont 34

IV. NIH TOOLBOX COGNITION BATTERY (CB): MEASURING LANGUAGE (VOCABULARY COMPREHENSION AND READING DECODING)
Richard C. Gershon, Jerry Slotkin, Jennifer J. Manly, David L. Blitz, Jennifer L. Beaumont, Deborah Schnipke, Kathleen Wallner-Allen, Roberta Michnick Golinkoff, Jean Berko Gleason, Kathy Hirsh-Pasek, Marilyn Jager Adams, and Sandra Weintraub 49

V. NIH TOOLBOX COGNITION BATTERY (CB): MEASURING WORKING MEMORY
David S. Tulsky, Noelle E. Carlozzi, Nicolas Chevalier, Kimberly A. Espy, Jennifer L. Beaumont, and Dan Mungas 70

VI. NIH TOOLBOX COGNITION BATTERY (CB): MEASURING PROCESSING SPEED
Noelle E. Carlozzi, David S. Tulsky, Robert V. Kail, and Jennifer L. Beaumont 88

VII. NIH TOOLBOX COGNITION BATTERY (CB): FACTOR STRUCTURE FOR 3 TO 15 YEAR OLDS
Dan Mungas, Keith Widaman, Philip David Zelazo, David Tulsky, Robert K. Heaton, Jerry Slotkin, David L. Blitz, and Richard C. Gershon 103

VIII. NIH TOOLBOX COGNITION BATTERY (CB): COMPOSITE SCORES OF CRYSTALLIZED, FLUID, AND OVERALL COGNITION
Natacha Akshoomoff, Jennifer L. Beaumont, Patricia J. Bauer, Sureyya S. Dikmen, Richard C. Gershon, Dan Mungas, Jerry Slotkin, David Tulsky, Sandra Weintraub, Philip David Zelazo, and Robert K. Heaton   119

IX. NIH TOOLBOX COGNITION BATTERY (CB): SUMMARY, CONCLUSIONS, AND IMPLICATIONS FOR COGNITIVE DEVELOPMENT
Patricia J. Bauer and Philip David Zelazo   133

APPENDIX A   147

COMMENTARY

COMMENTARY ON ZELAZO AND BAUER (EDITORS), NATIONAL INSTITUTES OF HEALTH TOOLBOX COGNITION BATTERY (CB): VALIDATION FOR CHILDREN BETWEEN 3 AND 15 YEARS
Nathan A. Fox   150

CONTRIBUTORS   156

STATEMENT OF EDITORIAL POLICY   164

SUBJECT INDEX   166

I. NIH TOOLBOX COGNITION BATTERY (CB): INTRODUCTION AND PEDIATRIC DATA*

Sandra Weintraub, Patricia J. Bauer, Philip David Zelazo, Kathleen Wallner-Allen, Sureyya S. Dikmen, Robert K. Heaton, David S. Tulsky, Jerry Slotkin, David L. Blitz, Noelle E. Carlozzi, Richard J. Havlik, Jennifer L. Beaumont, Dan Mungas, Jennifer J. Manly, Beth G. Borosh, Cindy J. Nowinski, and Richard C. Gershon

ABSTRACT This monograph presents the pediatric portion of the National Institutes of Health (NIH) Toolbox Cognition Battery (CB) of the NIH Toolbox for the Assessment of Neurological and Behavioral Function. The NIH Toolbox is an initiative of the Neuroscience Blueprint, a collaborative framework through which 16 NIH Institutes, Centers, and Offices jointly support neuroscience-related research, to accelerate discoveries and reduce the burden of nervous system disorders. The CB is one of four modules that measure cognitive, emotional, sensory, and motor health across the lifespan. The CB is unique in its continuity across childhood, adolescence, early adulthood, and old age, and in order to help create a common currency among disparate studies, it is also available at low cost to researchers for use in large-scale longitudinal and epidemiologic studies. This chapter describes the evolution of the CB; methods for selecting cognitive subdomains and instruments; the rationale for test design; and a validation study in children and adolescents, ages 3–15 years. Subsequent chapters feature detailed discussions of each test measure and its psychometric properties (Chapters 2–6), the factor structure of the test battery (Chapter 7), the effects of age and education on composite test scores (Chapter 8), and a final summary and discussion (Chapter 9). As the chapters in this monograph demonstrate, the CB has excellent psychometric properties, and the validation study provided evidence for the increasing differentiation of cognitive abilities with age.

Corresponding author: Sandra Weintraub, Cognitive Neurology and Alzheimer's Disease Center, Northwestern Feinberg School of Medicine, Chicago, IL, email: sweintraub@northwestern.edu

*This monograph was accepted under the editorship of W. Andrew Collins.

The NIH Toolbox was conceived as an instrument for the systematic collection of data on cognitive, emotional, sensory, and motor health across disparate studies. It was intended to provide a brief assessment tool for large-scale epidemiologic and longitudinal studies for projects in which neurologic function may not necessarily constitute the primary focus but in which its assessment could be useful and also allow cross-study comparisons. The NIH Toolbox was designed as part of the NIH Blueprint initiative in the neurosciences, involving 16 different institutes.[1] The Request for Applications from the NIH specified that the NIH Toolbox instruments: (1) include measures relevant to development and health across the life span from ages 3 to 85 years; (2) assess the full range of normal functioning (i.e., the instruments are not intended to screen for disease); (3) cover several different subdomains within each of four domains (cognitive, emotional, sensory, and motor) essential to health and life adaptation; (4) be brief and easy to administer and score; (5) be freely available to researchers; and (6) be modifiable to accommodate advances in science.

This monograph focuses on the development of the instruments in the NIH Toolbox that assess cognitive function—the Cognition Battery (CB). An initial challenge in meeting the mandate of the NIH Toolbox was the selection of particular subdomains for assessment. Cognition includes many essential subdomains, some of which require lengthy and complex methods of assessment, so difficult decisions needed to be made regarding which to include at the cost of others. A systematic, research-based process was followed to select the subdomains for assessment. The process resulted in a focus on (1) executive function and attention, (2) episodic memory, (3) language, (4) working memory, and (5) processing speed. In the first section of this chapter, we describe this process, explain how instruments were selected for the subdomains, and outline the steps taken to ensure the usability of the instruments for diverse populations.

A second significant challenge was creating a single set of measures that is valid and appropriate across the entire 3- to 85-year age range. The difficulty of achieving this goal was obvious at the outset from the lack of such measures in most areas of cognition (despite the need for such measures). More typically, constructs are measured with very different tasks at different ages. The second section of this chapter describes the steps taken to develop instruments that meet this goal of use across the lifespan. As discussed in more detail in Chapters 2–6, which are devoted to the individual instruments, some tests were borrowed from the adult literature and adapted for younger examinees, whereas others were selected from the child developmental literature and adapted for older examinees.

The final section of the chapter provides an introduction to a test for validation of the CB. The validation study included the full age range of the NIH Toolbox, ages 3–85 years, although this monograph focuses on the results of this study for children and young adolescents ages 3–15 years. The validation data from the younger and older adult populations will be published in a separate series of papers so that each population can be addressed in greater depth. To preview the conclusion: whereas the mandate to develop brief tasks to be used across the lifespan presented substantial challenges, it also afforded a significant opportunity to advance science by providing tools to further our understanding of cognitive function across the lifespan.

SUBDOMAIN SELECTION

The Cognition team was required to select the subdomains to be evaluated and then to determine the best measure of each subdomain. The selection of subdomains was based on: (1) their importance to the course of development and aging; (2) their significance for health and success in education and, in adults, for work; (3) their validation with respect to known underlying brain mechanisms; and (4) their ease of measurement and translation into brief test instruments. Evaluation of subdomains using these criteria was accomplished through widespread and reiterative input from multidisciplinary researchers and clinicians who specialize in different areas of cognitive functioning and who work with pediatric and/or adult populations. The first step was a survey of potential "end users" to determine the structure of the final NIH Toolbox and to identify subdomains to be assessed. The methods used to gather data and to establish consensus among potential NIH Toolbox end-users are detailed elsewhere (Gershon et al., 2010) and are only summarized here.

Research and clinical experts were identified via literature searches, from the Computer Retrieval of Information on Scientific Projects (CRISP) database (now known as the NIH Research Portfolio Online Reporting Tools [RePORT]), and/or by nomination by one of the 12 NIH science officers who comprised the NIH Toolbox Project Team at that time. Two Requests for Information (RFIs) were then solicited online from a total of 293 experts, and the RFIs were followed-up by telephone interviews of a subset of 44 experts. The information gathered from experts allowed us to identify cognitive domains ranked in order of their importance as judged by experts, and to determine the characteristics that would be desirable for the final instruments. The subdomains were ranked as follows: Executive function, episodic memory, language, processing speed, and attention. Table 1 shows the percentage of respondents ranking each of the sudomains among their top four subdomain rankings. Fifty-seven percent of respondents also listed a "general" or "global" cognitive score as desirable. The need for a global cognitive score was met through development of cognition composite scores, described in Chapter 8. Only 43% of respondents ranked visuospatial

TABLE 1

PERCENTAGE OF EXPERT RATERS ($N = 147$) RANKING SUBDOMAIN IN TOP 4

Subdomain	%
Executive function	95
Memory	93
General/global score	57
Language	55
Processing speed	52
Attention	50
Visuospatial function	43
Other 1	7
Other 2	3

© 2006–2012 National Institutes of Health and Northwestern University.

functions among their top four subdomains, so this subdomain was not included in the final list.

Searches of relevant databases in psychology and pediatrics were then conducted to review support for the selection of subdomains in terms of their importance for neurological and behavioral function, and to develop a test instrument library. The test instrument library was reviewed to determine whether there were existing instruments that would fulfill the needs of the NIH Toolbox. Meanwhile, large consensus meetings were held twice a year for the Steering Committee, consisting of all the NIH Toolbox major domain team leaders and NIH representatives, to evaluate the information gathered and make decisions about final choices. The Steering Committee also held monthly phone conferences to review progress. Below, each subdomain included in the final cognition battery is briefly described.

Executive Function and Attention

The subdomains of executive function (EF) and attention are described together because one of the EF measures is also a measure of selective attention. EF consists of a number of distinctive types of mental operations, subsumed by the term, "cognitive control," that are involved in the top-down modulation of goal-directed activity. Recent factor-analytic work with adults suggests that EF can be divided into three partially independent components: cognitive flexibility, inhibitory control, and working memory (Miyake et al., 2000). EF deficits are seen in patients with acquired focal damage to prefrontal cortex who experience profound impairment in behavioral regulation despite the preservation of many basic intellectual functions (see Stuss & Knight, 2002). In children, impairments in EF or delays in its development have been linked to attention deficit hyperactivity disorder (ADHD) (Doyle, 2006), autism spectrum disorders, Conduct Disorder, and other psychiatric conditions and symptoms.

Because of the importance of EF, the CB contains measures of all three components, although the measure of working memory is considered separately, below. The other measures (see Zelazo, Anderson, Richler, Wallner-Allen, & Beaumont, Chapter 2, this volume) include measures of cognitive flexibility (i.e., the ability to switch conceptual frameworks, measured by the Dimensional Change Card Sort; Zelazo, 2006), and a measure of inhibitory control (and selective attention), measured by a version of the Eriksen flanker task (Eriksen & Eriksen, 1974) that was adapted from the Attention Network Test (ANT; e.g., Rueda et al., 2004).

Episodic Memory

Episodic memory, the capacity for storing and retrieving information, is critical for the acquisition of knowledge and for building adaptive skills. This subdomain shows dramatic changes over the first two decades of life (see Bauer, Larkina, & Deocampo, 2011, for a review) and is also susceptible to a variety of diseases, including encephalitis and temporolimbic epilepsy, and, in adulthood, Alzheimer's disease (e.g., see Weintraub, Wicklund, & Salmon, 2012). Episodic memory for single object-specific actions is apparent in infants in the first year of life (e.g., Carver & Bauer, 1999). By the second year of life, infants remember temporally ordered sequences of items as well (e.g., Bauer, Wenner, Dropik, & Wewerka, 2000). In order to tap similar memory constructs in older children, adolescents, and adults for the CB, Bauer's (2007) imitation-based assessment of memory paradigm was modified to create the Toolbox Picture Sequence Memory Test (see Bauer et al., Chapter 3, this volume). This test is based on nonverbal pictorial stimuli that must be placed in a predefined sequence, with increasing numbers of pictures for older age groups.

Language

Language develops rapidly over the first 3 years of life, although further changes occur throughout childhood, and language proficiency is a fundamental skill that supports many other aspects of cognitive, social, and behavioral function. Indeed, when language development is delayed, the impact on further skill acquisition and academic progress can be profound (e.g., Dickinson, Golinkoff, & Hirsh-Pasek, 2010; Gleason & Ratner, 2009). Disorders such as dyslexia hinder otherwise talented individuals from achieving educational and career goals (e.g., Meisinger, Bloom, & Hynd, 2010; Ziegler et al., 2008).

Language consists of numerous components, including semantics, grammar, morphology, and phonology, and it is conveyed via multiple modalities including auditory comprehension, speaking, reading, and writing. Two aspects of language were selected for the CB, due in part to the ease with which they can be measured across the lifespan: auditory single word comprehension (i.e., receptive vocabulary) and single word reading aloud (oral reading recognition; see Gershon et al., Chapter 4, this volume). Auditory single word comprehension develops prior to overt speech usage in hearing individuals (Fenson et al., 1994). Vocabulary has been widely accepted as a surrogate measure for overall crystallized intelligence (Schmidt & Hunter, 2004). Oral reading proficiency also is a marker of educational opportunity in minority populations and can be used to adjust for group differences when comparing individuals of different ethnic and racial backgrounds (Manly, Byrd, Touradji, & Stern, 2004; Manly et al., 1999).

Working Memory

Although working memory is a component of executive function (e.g., Miyake et al., 2000), it is often studied on its own, or as a type of memory. From preschool age on, most working memory tasks either require retaining and reorganizing items before recalling them (e.g., backward digit span task), or completing some processing activity in between presentations of the to-be-recalled items (e.g., listening span task). Such tasks tap into both information processing and storage, and yield a measure of working memory span that corresponds to the maximal amount of accurately recalled information. Working memory shows age-related improvements across childhood (as well as age-related declines during senescence). Like executive function more broadly, working memory depends on prefrontal cortex, and is vulnerable to disruption from a wide range of cerebral insults (see Tulsky et al., Chapter 5, this volume).

Processing Speed

Processing speed (PS), which refers to the speed with which simple cognitive operations can be performed, was included in the CB because it is very sensitive to any form of cerebral insult (see DeLuca & Kalmar, 2007; Weiler, Forbes, Kirkwood, & Waber, 2003) and to changes in development (e.g., Kail, 1991). Although PS paradigms often are based on motor reaction time, Sternberg's (1966) elegant paradigm demonstrated that mental processing time can be separated from motor response time, and that it varies with the number of mental operations required by a given task. The construct represented in the CB is the simple reaction time required to make a same-different comparison between two visually presented stimuli (see Carlozzi, Tulsky, Kail, & Beaumont, Chapter 6, this volume).

INSTRUMENT SELECTION

Following identification of the cognitive subdomains, additional experts were recruited to help develop tests. These experts held weekly conference calls to review decisions, update progress, and assure consistency of methods across all subdomains. Individual subdomain teams were also formed and these teams convened as needed to work on their specific tests. In addition to the Steering Committee meetings and conference calls, the entire CB team held a day-long meeting in July, 2007, to determine the particular instruments to be subjected to validation testing. During that meeting, the CB team derived criteria for validation studies, including acceptable levels of test–retest reliability and convergent and discriminant validity. In 2008, a public conference was held in Bethesda, Maryland, to present the NIH Toolbox to an expert advisory panel and obtain feedback. Written critiques of the subdomains and instruments were reviewed by the CB team and addressed. In 2010, we conducted several conference calls with 16 expert consultants to present the version of the CB created for validation testing and to invite feedback prior to initiating the validation study.

The general principles that guided decision-making regarding the NIH Toolbox instruments were:

1. *Versatility*: Measures should be capable of monitoring neurological and behavioral health status and function over time (as in longitudinal epidemiological studies), and capable of evaluating effectiveness of interventions and treatments (as in clinical trials). Instruments should be readily portable from one type of study design to another and have minimal ceiling and floor effects.
2. *Brevity*: Measures should be brief, to ensure low respondent burden. The targeted total time for the CB was 30 min (ages 7–85 years), and 20 min for children from 3 to 6 years of age.
3. *Methodological Soundness*: Measures should demonstrate validity and reliability.
4. *Dynamic*: Measures should be internally flexible (e.g., adaptive testing), and instruments should demonstrate sensitivity to change over time.
5. *State-of-the-art design*: Measures should employ modern psychometric approaches to the measurement of latent dimensions (e.g., item response theory models and computer-adaptive testing, to the extent relevant).

6. *Diversity*: Measures should have known properties across cultures and age ranges. English and Spanish versions should be developed and validated in culturally and geographically diverse groups.

In addition to these features, the instruments were submitted to scrutiny for their adaptability to the key populations that were to be assessed using the NIH Toolbox. Four special working groups were convened to examine the constructs selected and the instruments and procedures being developed with consideration of people from different ethnic, racial, and cultural backgrounds; the needs of older adults; the needs of people with disabilities; and the needs of children. These working groups were made up of project scientists and external consultants. Each group reviewed the instruments and procedures being developed from its particular perspective and identified areas of concern and proposed ways to address those concerns. The working groups held meetings and conference calls, discussed issues within groups, and sometimes partnered with each other when similar issues arose. Each group provided recommendations to the Cognition team, as well as to the Emotional, Sensation, and Motor teams, on ways to enhance the usability and relevance of the NIH Toolbox for diverse populations from ages 3 to 85 years.

The Cultural Working Group strived to ensure that the measures were culturally sensitive and conceptually appropriate across different cultures and languages. For example, they made recommendations for wording changes, picture changes, and suggested guidelines for determining language proficiency. The Geriatric Working Group and the Accessibility Working Group addressed issues relating to the suitability of instruments for those with motor and sensory impairments, often seen in the elderly, and for those with other impairments related to disability. Issues such as font size, image size, type of motoric response required, and color of stimuli (with respect to color blindness) were considered within the context of working to increase the accessibility of tasks for those in the general US population with a disability. The Pediatric Working Group addressed the difficulties of designing instruments suitable for use with young children. Because the work of this group was most relevant to the pediatric data reported here, we discuss it more fully.

Developing instruments for use across the broad age range of 3–85 years presented significant challenges. Children differ from adults in many ways, including social, emotional, and selfregulatory ways that may affect performance on tasks designed to measure cognition. A major challenge was to structure tasks and the testing environment so that differences in task performance across different ages would more likely reflect differences in competence for the construct of interest rather than differences in other performance factors. For example, children are able to demonstrate competence for constructs at younger ages when simple, easy-to-follow instructions are used and when task materials are engaging, concrete, and familiar. In addition, compared to healthy young adults, most children and even adolescents have shorter attention spans, are more easily distracted by external stimuli, and are less proficient at regulating their attention, behavior, and level of motivation to the task at hand.

In consideration of the challenges of measurement in children in particular, the Pediatric Working Group developed a set of pediatric assessment principles to inform instrument design and to standardize assessment procedures across all NIH Toolbox instruments. These principles addressed instrument design characteristics, the testing environment, the psychological and physical needs of the child, and the nature and extent of the interactions among the test administrator, the child, and the parent (where appropriate). For example, it was considered important to use simple instructions, have practice trials to ensure understanding, establish stop rules to minimize failure experiences, and have an examiner present during testing. The Pediatric Working group reviewed all NIH Toolbox instruments and considered whether each was age appropriate, assessed an appropriate construct, was appropriately sized, and was nonthreatening. The Pediatric Working Group advocated for building flexibility into the computer interface (e.g., the ability to repeat instructions) and made recommendations for an appropriate response mechanism (e.g., touchscreen, mouse). Recommendations were also made on whether task instructions should be "live" or "prerecorded" and provided by computer to standardize presentation and, when it was decided to use a prerecorded voice, the group consulted on what the quality of the voice and the gender of the speaker should be. The guidance provided by the Pediatric Working Group, as well as the other working groups, significantly improved the NIH Toolbox overall and strengthened its ability to obtain valid assessments from diverse populations—not just from children.

VALIDATION STUDY

To determine the reliability and validity of the instruments as measures of the target subdomains, the Cognition team conducted a validation study involving a total of 476 participants recruited from multiple sites (Chicago's NorthShore University HealthSystems, Emory University in Atlanta, New Jersey's Kessler Institute for Rehabilitation, and the University of Minnesota). Eligible participants were 3–85 years of age and sample recruitment was distributed across age, gender, race, and education strata. Table 2 illustrates the pediatric validation sample, including the 208 three- to fifteen year olds whose data are featured in this monograph. There were a total of one hundred twenty 120 three- to six year olds and 88 eight- to fifteen year olds. As

TABLE 2

VALIDATION PEDIATRIC SAMPLE DEMOGRAPHICS ($N = 208$)

Age Groups	Level of Parents' Education	Gender		Race/Ethnicity		
		Male	Female	White	Black	Hispanic/Other/ Multiple Races
3–6 years	<High School	6	5	5	5	1
$N = 120$	High School Graduate	29	27	23	19	14
	College Graduate+	29	24	26	16	11
Total		64	56	54	40	26
8–15 years	<High School	4	6	4	5	1
$N = 88$	High School Graduate	22	23	18	13	14
	College Graduate+	14	19	16	7	10
Total		40	48	38	25	25

© 2006–2012 National Institutes of Health and Northwestern University.

Table 3 indicates, not all ages were sampled in this study; also, education levels indicated in the table are defined as highest parental education. A subset of 66 child participants (approximately 32%) completed a retest 7–21 days later to assess test–retest reliability and practice effects.

Validation Measures

Validation measures were selected by reviewing published tests commonly used in neuropsychological practice to assess the constructs being tapped by the CB tests. Table 3 shows each CB measure and its associated validation measures. Table 4 shows CB measures and the validation measures by age group to which each was administered. Table 5 shows a sample of the criterion grid established for judging validity, using the measure of working memory (The NIH Toolbox List Sorting Working Memory Test) as an example.

Pearson correlation coefficients between age and test performance were calculated separately for children and adults to describe the developmental and aging-related associations for each measure. Intraclass correlation coefficients (ICC) were calculated to evaluate test–retest reliability. Across measures, $ICC < .4$ were considered poor, .4 to .74 were considered adequate and $\geq .75$ were considered excellent. Convergent validity was assessed with correlations between each Toolbox measure and a well-established validation measure of the same construct. Across measures, $r < .3$ were considered poor, .3 to .59 were considered adequate, and $\geq .6$ were considered excellent. Evidence of discriminant validity consisted of lower correlations with selected validation measures of a *different* cognitive construct. The rationale for selection of each validation instrument is discussed in the context of the individual chapters of the monograph.

TABLE 3

COGNITION BATTERY (CB) AND CORRESPONDING CONVERGENT VALIDATION MEASURES FOR CHILDREN

Cognition Subdomain	NIH Toolbox CB Measures	Validation Measure
Executive Function	Flanker Inhibitory Control and Attention Test	WPPSI-III Block Design (3–6 years)
	Dimensional Change Card Sort Test	D-KEFS Color Word Interference (8–15 years)
Episodic Memory	Picture Sequence Memory Test	NEPSY-II Sentence Repetition (3–6 years)
		Rey Auditory-Verbal Learning Test (RAVLT; 3-trial version; 8–15 years)[a]
		Brief Visuospatial Memory Test-Revised (BVMT-R; 8–15 years)[a]
Language	Picture Vocabulary Test	Peabody Picture Vocabulary Test 4th Edition (PPVT-IV)
	Oral Reading Recognition Test	Wide Range Achievement Test 4th Edition (WRAT-IV) Reading Subtest
Working Memory	List Sorting Working Memory Test	NEPSY-II Sentence Repetition (3–6 years)
		WISC-IV Letter Number Sequencing (8–15 years)
Processing Speed	Pattern Comparison Processing Speed Test	WPPSI-III or WISC-IV Processing Speed Composite, as appropriate
		Paced Auditory Serial Addition Test (PASAT; 8–15 years)

Note. WPPSI-III, Wechsler Preschool and Primary Scale of Intelligence, 3rd Edition; D-KEFS, Delis–Kaplan Executive Function Scales; NEPSY-II, Developmental Neuropsychological Assessment Battery, 2nd Edition; WISC-IV, Wechsler Intelligence Scale for Children, 4th Edition.
[a]Two validation measures were used in order to capture both verbal and visuospatial memory.

PLAN FOR THE REST OF THE MONOGRAPH

Chapters 2–6 each addresses a single subdomain. In each chapter, we review the rationale for inclusion of that subdomain in the battery, and the importance of that subdomain for health. We also review the literature on developmental changes in the subdomain throughout childhood and into adolescence, and the evidence linking the subdomain or construct to brain functioning. The test instruments are described in greater detail, including the adaptations to enable testing across the 3–85 years age range. We present results of a validation study and describe the psychometric properties of the new CB measures. Chapter 7 of the monograph reports the results of a

TABLE 4
NIH Toolbox Cognition Battery (CB) and Validation Measures by Age Cohort

	3–4	5–6	8–15	20–85
NIH Toolbox CB Measures				
Dimensional Change Card Sort Test	Yes	Yes	Yes	Yes
Flanker Inhibitory Control and Attention Test	Yes	Yes	Yes	Yes
Picture Sequence Memory Test	Yes	Yes	Yes	Yes
List Sorting Working Memory Test	Yes	Yes	Yes	Yes
Pattern Comparison Processing Speed Test	Yes	Yes	Yes	Yes
Oral Reading Recognition Test	Yes	Yes	Yes	Yes
Picture Vocabulary Test	Yes	Yes	Yes	Yes
Validation Measures				
Wisconsin Card Sort Test-64 cards			Yes	Yes
Paced Auditory Serial Addition Test			Yes	Yes
EXAMINER Dot Counting Test			Yes	Yes
Delis–Kaplan Executive Function: Color/Word Interference			Yes	Yes
Rey Auditory Verbal Learning Test			Yes	Yes
Brief Visual Memory Test-Revised			Yes	Yes
Wide Range Achievement Test-IV Reading	Yes	Yes	Yes	Yes
Peabody Picture Vocabulary Test-IV	Yes	Yes	Yes	Yes
NEPSY-II				
Sentence Repetition	Yes	Yes		
Speeded Naming	Yes	Yes		
WPPSI–III				
Block Design	Yes	Yes		
Coding		Yes		
Symbol Search		Yes		
WISC-IV				
Coding			Yes	
Letter-Number Sequencing			Yes	
Symbol Search			Yes	
WAIS-IV				
Coding				Yes
Letter-Number Sequencing				Yes
Symbol Search				Yes
Questionnaires				
Child Behavior Questionnaire	Yes	Yes		
Sociodemographics Form-Parent	Yes	Yes	Yes	
Sociodemographics Form-Subject				Yes
Cognitive Information Form	Yes	Yes	Yes	Yes

Note. NINDS EXAMINER: National Institute of Neurological Diseases and Stroke battery of "Domain Specific Test of Executive Function," http://examiner.ucsf.edu/index.htm; NEPSY-II, Developmental Neuropsychological Assessment Battery, 2nd Edition; WPPSI-III, Wechsler Preschool and Primary Scale of Intelligence, 3rd Edition; WISC-IV, Wechsler Intelligence Scale for Children, 4th Edition; WAIS-IV, Wechsler Adult Scale of Intelligence, 4th Edition.

NIH TOOLBOX COGNITION BATTERY (CB)

TABLE 5
Sample Criteria for Validation of Toolbox List Sorting Working Memory Test; One List, Two List, and Total Scores

Analysis	Criterion
Measure-level selection criteria	
Convergent validity (NEPSY-II Sentence Repetition; WISC-IV Letter Number Sequencing) by age band and overall	Minimum correlation of .5
Divergent validity: PPVT-IV, D-KEFS Color Word Interference, WCST-64	.1 *less than* correlation with others
Test–Retest Reliability (*ICC*)	.5
Correlation between One List and Two List	.75
Internal Consistency Reliability (Split-half)	.65
Internal Consistency Reliability (alpha)	.55
Age effects	*r*-Squared approx. .2; linear effect through childhood; ages 20–35 stable (highest functioning); >age 35 declining; from middle age on, *r*-squared again approx. .2
Demographic effects (education, ethnicity, & gender) by age	Education: Linear relation for adults (*r*-squared approx. .1); for children, age and education will be highly correlated (just look at age)
Floor/ceiling effects	No evidence of floor or ceiling effects
Test timing by age band and overall	5 min
Primary test score means stratified separately on demographic variables (education, ethnicity, and gender)	No differential functioning (significant differences) between referent and focal groups
Percent of respondents making it to an item	Same as frequency pattern for total score
Item-level selection criteria	
Item-total correlations	Should range .15–.40 (should covary with *p*-value)
Item *p*values	*p*-Values should range .15–.95

Note. PPVT-IV, Peabody Picture Vocabulary Test-4th Edition; WISC-IV, Wechsler Intelligence Scale for Children, 4th Edition; NEPSY-II, Developmental Neuropsychological Assessment, 2nd Edition; D-KEFS, Delis-Kaplan Executive Function Scales; WCST-64, Wisconsin Card Sorting Test-64 Card version.

confirmatory factor analysis of the CB validation study. Chapter 8 reports the creation of CB composite scores and the relations of demographic variables to these scores. The final chapter provides brief summaries of the rationale for development of the CB and the major findings from the validation study, followed by discussion of the implications of the NIH Toolbox CB for the study of cognitive development, the limitations of the battery, and directions for further development of the instrument.

REFERENCES

Bauer, P. J. (2007). *Remembering the times of our lives: Memory in infancy and beyond.* Mahwah, NJ: Erlbaum.

Bauer, P. J., Larkina, M., & Deocampo, J. (2011). Early memory development. In U. Goswami (Ed.), *The Wiley-Blackwell handbook of childhood cognitive development* (2nd ed., pp. 153–179). Oxford, UK: Wiley-Blackwell.

Bauer, P. J., Wenner, J. A., Dropik, P. L., & Wewerka, S. S. (2000). Parameters of remembering and forgetting in the transition from infancy to early childhood. *Monographs of the Society for Research in Child Development,* **65**(4), i–vi, 1–204.

Brocki, K., Fan, J., & Fossella, J. (2008). Placing neuroanatomical models of executive function in a developmental context: Imaging and imaging–genetic strategies. *Annals of the New York Academy of Sciences,* **1129**, 246–255.

Carver, L. J., & Bauer, P. J. (1999). When the event is more than the sum of its parts: Nine-month-olds' long-term ordered recall. *Memory,* **7**, 147–174.

DeLuca, J., & Kalmar, J. H. (2007). *Information processing speed in clinical populations.* London: Psychology Press.

Dickinson, D. K., Golinkoff, R. M., & Hirsh-Pasek, K. (2010). Speaking out for language: Why language is central to reading development. *Educational Researcher,* **39**(4), 305–310.

Doyle, A. E. (2006). Executive functions in attention-deficit/hyperactivity disorder. *Journal of Clinical Psychiatry,* **67** (Suppl 8), 21–26.

Eriksen, B. A., & Eriksen, C. W. (1974). Effects of noise letters upon the identification of a target letter in a nonsearch task. *Perception and Psychophysics,* **16**, 143–149.

Fenson, L., Dale, P. S., Reznick, J. S., Bates, E., Thal, D. J., & Pethick, S. J. (1994). Variability in early communicative development. *Monographs of the Society for Research in Child Development,* **59**, 1–173.

Gershon, R. C., Cella, D., Fox, N. A., Havlik, R. J., Hendrie, H. C., & Wagster, M. V. (2010). Assessment of neurological and behavioural function: The NIH Toolbox. *Lancet Neurology,* **9**(2), 138–139.

Gleason, J. B., & Ratner, N. B. (Eds.). (2009). *The development of language* (7th ed.). Boston: Pearson/Allyn & Bacon.

Kail, R. (1991). Processing time declines exponentially during childhood and adolescence. *Developmental Psychology,* **27**, 259–266.

Manly, J. J., Byrd, D. A., Touradji, P., & Stern, Y. (2004). Acculturation, reading level, and neuropsychological test performance among African American elders. *Applied Neuropsychology,* **11**(1), 37–46.

Manly, J. J., Jacobs, D. M., Sano, M., Bell, K., Merchant, C. A., Small, S. A., et al. (1999). Effect of literacy on neuropsychological test performance in nondemented, education-matched elders. *Journal of the International Neuropsychological Society,* **5**(3), 191–202.

Meisinger, E. B., Bloom, J. S., & Hynd, G. W. (2010). Reading fluency: Implications for the assessment of children with reading disabilities. *Annals of Dyslexia,* **60**(1), 1–17.

Miyake, A., Friedman, N. P., Emerson, M. J., Witzki, A. H., Howerter, A., & Wager, T. D. (2000). The unity and diversity of executive functions and their contributions to complex "frontal lobe" tasks: A latent variable analysis. *Cognitive Psychology,* **41**, 49–100.

NICHD Early Child Care Research Network. (2005). *Child care and child development: Results from the NICHD Study of Early Child Care and Youth Development.* New York: Guilford Publications.

Rueda, M. R., Fan, J., McCandliss, B. D., Halparin, J. D., Gruber, D. B., Lercari, L. P., et al. (2004). Development of attentional networks in childhood. *Neuropsychologia,* **42**, 1029–1040.

Schmidt, F. L., & Hunter, J. (2004). General mental ability in the world of work: Occupational attainment and job performance. *Journal of Personality and Social Psychology,* **86**(1), 162–173.

Shaywitz, S. E., Shaywitz, B. A., Fulbright, R. K., Skudlarski, P., Mencl, W. E., Constable, R. T., et al. (2003). Neural systems for compensation and persistence: Young adult outcome of childhood reading disability. *Biological Psychiatry,* **54**(1), 25–33.

Sternberg, S. (1966). High-speed scanning in human memory. *Science,* **153**, 652–654.

Weiler, M. D., Forbes, P., Kirkwood, M., & Waber, D. (2003). The developmental course of processing speed in children with and without learning disabilities. *Journal of Experimental Child Psychology,* **85**(2), 178–194.

Weintraub, S., Wicklund, A. H., & Salmon, D. P. (2012). The neuropsychological profile of Alzheimer disease. In D. Selkoe, D. Holzman, & E. Mandelkow (Eds.), *The biology of Alzheimer's Disease* (pp. 25–52). Woodbury, NY: Cold Spring Harbor Laboratory Press.

Zelazo, P. D. (2006). The Dimensional Change Card Sort (DCCS): A method of assessing executive function in children. *Nature Protocols,* **1**, 297–301.

Ziegler, J. C., Castel, C., Pech-Georgel, C., George, F., Alario, F. X., & Perry, C. (2008). Developmental dyslexia and the dual route model of reading: Simulating individual differences and subtypes. *Cognition,* **107**(1), 151–178.

NOTE

1. These institutes are: National Institute on Aging (NIA), National Institute on Mental Health (NIMH), National Institute on Drug Abuse (NIDA), National Institute on Neurological Disorders & Stroke (NINDS), National Institute on Environmental Health Sciences (NIEHS), National Institute on Deafness and Other Communicative Disorders (NIDCD), National Eye Institute (NEI), National Institute on Child Health and Human Development (NICHD), National Institute of Nursing Research (NINR), National Institute on General Medical Sciences (NIGMS), Office of Behavioral and Social Sciences Research (OBSSR), National Center on Complementary and Alternative Medicine (NCCAM), National Institute on Alcohol Abuse and Alcoholism (NIAAA), National Center on Research Resources (NCRR).

II. NIH TOOLBOX COGNITION BATTERY (CB): MEASURING EXECUTIVE FUNCTION AND ATTENTION

Philip David Zelazo, Jacob E. Anderson, Jennifer Richler, Kathleen Wallner-Allen, Jennifer L. Beaumont, and Sandra Weintraub

ABSTRACT In this chapter, we discuss two measures designed to assess executive function (EF) as part of the NIH Toolbox Cognition Battery (CB) and report pediatric data from the validation study. EF refers to the goal-directed cognitive control of thought, action, and emotion. Two measures were adapted for standardized computer administration: the Dimensional Change Card Sort (a measure of cognitive flexibility) and a flanker task (a measure of inhibitory control in the context of selective visual attention). Results reveal excellent developmental sensitivity across childhood, excellent reliability, and (in most cases) excellent convergent validity. Correlations between the new NIH Toolbox measures and age were higher for younger children (3–6 years) than for older children (8–15 years), and evidence of increasing differentiation of EF from other aspects of cognition (indexed by receptive vocabulary) was obtained.

In this chapter, we discuss two measures designed to assess executive function (EF) and the closely related construct of executive attention as part of the NIH Toolbox Cognition Battery (CB).

Subdomain Definition

In its broadest sense, the term "attention" refers to the allocation of information processing toward a stimulus or stimuli, but the term is typically used in a more narrow fashion to refer to the allocation of a particular type of information processing, namely that which requires limited conscious resources. According to one well-supported taxonomy, attention is usefully described in terms of three general functions—alerting, orienting, and executive attention—that draw differentially on

---

Corresponding author: Philip David Zelazo, Institute of Child Development, University of Minnesota, 51 East River Road, Minneapolis, MN 55455-0345, email: zelazo@umn.edu

three subsets of a large-scale, distributed network in the brain that includes frontal areas, basal ganglia, parts of parietal cortex, and the anterior cingulate cortex (Fan, McCandliss, Sommer, Raz, & Posner, 2002; Posner & Boies, 1971; see Raz & Buhle, 2006, for review). The construct of executive attention, which encompasses endogenous attentional processes that are under cognitive control, overlaps considerably with the construct of executive function (EF), also called cognitive control. EF corresponds to the deliberate, top-down neurocognitive processes involved in the conscious, goal-directed control of thought, action, and emotion, and it involves processes such as cognitive flexibility, inhibitory control, and working memory. Like executive attention, EF depends on the integrity of prefrontal cortex (PFC), and appears to develop most rapidly during the preschool years, together with the rapid growth of neural networks involving PFC, although it is now clear that executive attention, EF, and PFC all continue to develop into adolescence and beyond (Zelazo, Carlson, & Kesek, 2008). Measures of executive attention, such as the Eriksen Flanker task (Eriksen & Eriksen, 1974) are also considered measures of EF.

Importance During Childhood

There is currently widespread interest in the development of EF, which is increasingly recognized as a major influence on key developmental outcomes. Moffit et al. (2011), for example, found that EF in childhood predicts (as a gradient) physical health, substance dependence, socioeconomic status, and the likelihood of a criminal conviction at age 32 years, even after controlling for social class of origin and IQ. Impairments in EF are a prominent feature of numerous clinical conditions with childhood onset, including Attention Deficit/Hyperactivity Disorder (ADHD) and autism, but research suggests that EF is surprisingly malleable in childhood (e.g., Diamond, Barnett, Thomas, & Munro, 2007; Rueda, Posner, & Rothbart, 2005), and indeed, the beneficial effects of interventions targeting social and emotional learning have been found to be mediated, in large part, by experience-induced improvements in EF (Riggs, Greenberg, Kusche, & Pentz, 2006). Emerging research also suggests that EF may be a better predictor than IQ of school readiness and academic achievement (e.g., Blair & Razza, 2007; Eigsti et al., 2006), and teachers often report that the most important determinant of classroom success in kindergarten and early grades is the extent to which children can sit still, pay attention, and follow rules (e.g., McClelland et al., 2007).

A major challenge in research on EF has been methodological: the absence of measures that are suitable from early childhood through adulthood. EF is an effortful process required for solving relatively novel, challenging problems, and most measures of EF used with young children, such as the standard version of the Dimensional Change Card Sort (DCCS; Zelazo, 2006) or the Less Is More task (Carlson, Davis, & Leach, 2005), are too easy for (most) older children and adults. In contrast, many classic neuropsychological measures of EF, such as the Wisconsin Card Sorting Test (Grant & Berg, 1948) or the Color-Word Stroop task (Stroop, 1935), are either too difficult for young children or inappropriate for other reasons (e.g., the Stroop task assumes not only that participants be literate, but also that reading be fully automatized). The absence of common measures has made it difficult to characterize the lifespan development of EF—for example, to determine whether the development of EF occurs more rapidly during the preschool years or during the transition to adolescence. This type of comparison requires a common metric of developmental change during both periods, together with scores that are commensurable and can be mapped onto that common metric.

The absence of a single measure of EF that can be used across a wide age range in childhood has also made it difficult to determine whether, and if so how, the relation between EF and other aspects of cognitive function changes with age. Research on the structure of cognition, and the extent to which this structure develops, is important for a general understanding of the nature of cognitive development. Whereas some accounts suggest that a good deal of cognitive structure is a consequence of evolutionary adaptations and present at birth (e.g., see chapters in Hirschfeld & Gelman, 1994), other accounts emphasize the role of individual experiences during ontogeny (e.g., see chapters in Roberts, 2007). According to the Interactive Specialization model (e.g., Johnson & Munakata, 2005), for example, neurocognitive development in general involves the increasing functional specialization of neural systems that are initially relatively undifferentiated but that become more specialized (or modularized) as a function of experience.

A pattern of functional specialization may characterize the structure of EF itself. Factor-analytic work with adults is consistent with the suggestion that EF is a hierarchical construct that is characterized by both unity and diversity (Miyake et al., 2000), such that performance on measures of EF in adults can be captured by three partially independent latent variables, reflecting cognitive flexibility, inhibitory control, and working memory (Miyake et al., 2000). Research with younger participants, however, is generally consistent with a single-factor solution (Wiebe, Espy, & Charack, 2008; Wiebe et al., 2011), although several studies have found that the Miyake et al. (2000) model provides a good account of children's performance by middle childhood (Lehto, Juujärvi, Kooistra, & Pulkkinen, 2003; McAuley & White, 2011; Visu-Petra, Benga, & Miclea, 2007). It is possible, therefore, that EF becomes differentiated with age, although the use of different measures as different ages makes this possibility difficult to assess.

Toolbox Measurement

In order to provide a relatively comprehensive assessment of EF across the lifespan, the NIHTB-CB was designed to include measures of cognitive flexibility and inhibitory control, as well as a measure of working memory, considered separately (see Tulsky et al., Chapter 5, this volume). Together, these three measures capture all aspects of EF identified by the most differentiated, tripartite model of EF (Miyake et al., 2000), and the NIHTB-CB can therefore be used to trace developmental changes in the relation among aspects of EF (with the caveat that there is only one measure per aspect), as well as changes in the relation between EF and other domains of cognition.

The selected measure of inhibitory control has the distinct advantage that it also provides a measure of executive attention (Fan et al., 2002). More precisely, the measure of inhibitory control (considered as an aspect of EF) can also be interpreted as a measure of executive attention (considered as an aspect of attention).

As a consequence of the initial process of measure selection described by Weintraub et al. (Chapter 1, this volume), one measure each of two aspects of EF, cognitive flexibility and inhibitory control/executive attention, emerged as candidates that were freely available (in the public domain) and that had the potential to be modified, in an iterative fashion, to meet the initial usability objectives of the NIH Toolbox—namely, that they be computer-administered, brief, and suitable for participants between the ages 3 and 85 years. These measures were then subjected to an iterative process of measure development that included pilot testing and a "prevalidation" study. This process involved modifying existing measures in order to satisfy the criteria of the Pediatric (and Geriatric), Accessibility, and Cultural Working Groups (see Weintraub et al., Chapter 1, this volume). For example, measures were modified so that the instructions were easy to understand and would translate readily into Spanish, the visual displays were engaging for all participants, and the number of trials in each task was minimized while maximizing test–retest reliability and validity.

Executive Function-Cognitive Flexibility

The Dimensional Change Card Sort (DCCS) was selected as the measure of cognitive flexibility, also known as task switching or set shifting. This task, designed by Zelazo and colleagues (Frye, Zelazo, & Palfai, 1995; Zelazo, 2006) based on Luria's seminal work on rule use, has been used extensively to study the development of EF in childhood, and indeed, it may be the most widely used measure of EF in young children (Beck, Schaefer, Pang, & Carlson, 2011). In the standard version of the DCCS, children are shown two target cards (e.g., a blue rabbit and a red boat) and asked to sort a series of bivalent test cards (e.g., red rabbits and blue boats) first according to one dimension (e.g., color), and then according to the other (e.g., shape). Most 3 year olds perseverate during the postswitch phase, continuing to sort test cards by the first dimension, whereas most 5 year olds switch flexibly (e.g., Dick, Overton, & Kovacs, 2005; Kirkham, Cruess, & Diamond, 2003; Zelazo, Müller, Frye, & Marcovitch, 2003). In a study comparing 3 and 5 year olds, Moriguchi and Hiraki (2009) used near-infrared spectroscopy (NIRS) to measure the concentration of oxygenated haemoglobin (oxy-Hb) in ventrolateral prefrontal cortex during performance on this task. Following presentation of the test cards, both 5 year olds and those 3 year olds who switched flexibly on the task showed an increase in oxy-Hb bilaterally, whereas 3 year olds who failed the task did not. More challenging versions of this task have also been used with older children, adolescents, and young and old adults (Diamond & Kirkham, 2005; Morton, Bosma, & Ansari, 2009; Zelazo, Craik, & Booth, 2004; see Zelazo, 2006). Both the standard version of this task and a more challenging version show excellent test–retest reliability in childhood ($ICCs = .90-.94$; Beck et al., 2011).

Executive Function-Inhibitory Control and Attention

A version of the Eriksen flanker task (Eriksen & Eriksen, 1974) was adapted from the Attention Network Test (ANT; e.g., Rueda et al., 2004). In a flanker task, participants are required to indicate the left–right orientation of a centrally presented stimulus while inhibiting attention to the potentially incongruent stimuli that surround it (i.e., the flankers, two on either side). In the traditional flanker task, the stimuli are arrows pointing left or right, whereas in the ANT version used with children, the stimuli are fish (designed to be more engaging and also larger, which makes the task easier). The version created for the CB includes both an easier fish block and a more difficult arrows block. On some trials, the orientation of the flanking stimuli is congruent with the orientation of the central stimulus, and on others it is incongruent. Performance on the incongruent trials provides a measure of inhibitory control in the context of visual selective attention (which can also be considered a measure of executive attention).

To assess the construct validity of the new EF and attention measures for participants between the ages of 3 and 15 years, we examined data from the validation study of the CB and compared performance on the Toolbox DCCS Test and the Toolbox Flanker Inhibitory Control and Attention Test to performance on several established instruments (i.e., validation measures). We predicted that the CB measures would show excellent convergent validity with relevant validation measures, as well as adequate discriminant validity, shown by lower correlations with receptive vocabulary than with appropriate convergent measures. In addition, however, we expected that there would be less evidence of discriminant validity among younger children. This expectation was based upon the hypothesis that EF and attention become increasing differentiated from other aspects of cognition as a function of experience-dependent neural specialization.

METHOD

Participants

As described below, data from some of the 208 participants in the validation study (see Weintraub et al., Chapter 1, this volume; Table 3) were missing or excluded from the final analyses (e.g., for failing to reach criterion during practice trials), leaving final samples that ranged from $n = 166–188$ for each measure.

Measures

Toolbox Dimensional Change Card Sort (DCCS) Test

The modified version of this task included in the CB consisted of four blocks: practice, preswitch, postswitch, and mixed. In the practice block, participants were given a series of practice trials in which they were shown pictorial stimuli on a touch screen monitor, and instructed to match centrally presented test stimuli to one of two lateralized target stimuli (see Figure 1 for

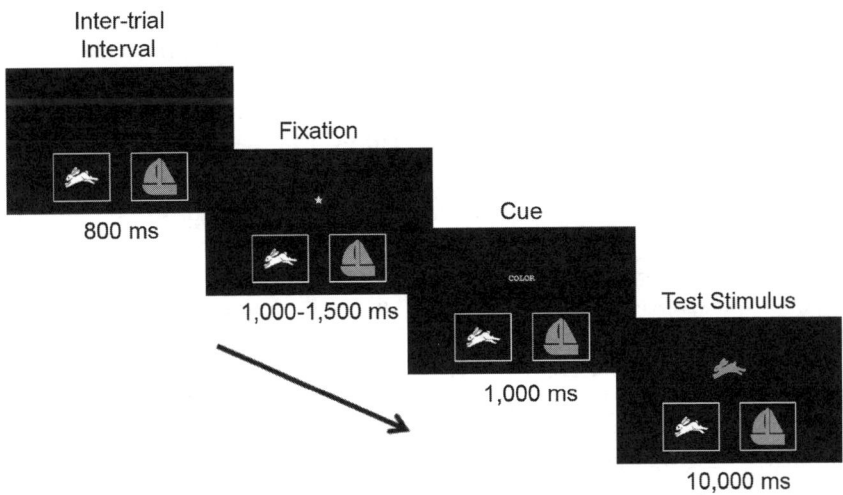

FIGURE 1.—Trial sequence for the Toolbox Dimensional Change Card Sort Test (with practice stimuli). © 2006–2012 National Institutes of Health and Northwestern University.

the trial structure and the timing of each stimulus). Target stimuli were a white rabbit and a green boat. Bivalent test stimuli included a green rabbit and a white boat. Participants were instructed to match (sort) either by shape or by color (counterbalanced across participants) by touching the target stimulus that matched the test stimulus on the relevant dimension. In the validation study, a touch screen monitor was used to record participants' responses, although subsequent research suggests that a simple key press (i.e., using keys that are spatially congruent with the target stimuli) works equally well at all ages. Instructions appeared visually on the monitor and were also read aloud by the experimenter to all children under age 8 years. On each trial, for participants who received shape first, (1) the word "shape" was presented both visually and auditorily (via a recording) on each trial, (2) a test stimulus appeared on the screen for up to 10,000 msec, (3) participants responded by touching one of the two target stimuli, which cancelled the test stimulus, and (4) participants were given feedback about their responses. Children were required to get three out of four practice trials correct, and if they failed, the four practice trials were repeated up to three times. Once they met this criterion, they received a comparable series of practice trials for the other dimension (color, in this example). Children who met criterion for each dimension proceeded to the test trials, which were similar in structure but involved different shapes and colors and no feedback. Two children failed to meet criterion, and no data were collected from these children. Test trials started with a preswitch block that consisted of five trials in which children were instructed to sort by the last dimension used in the practice block (color, in this example). The trial structure and the timing of each stimulus was the same as in the practice block. No feedback was provided on test trials. Children had to get four out of five trials correct to proceed to the next block, which consisted of five trials in which children were instructed to sort by the other dimension (shape, in this example). The transition between blocks was noted explicitly by instructions to switch. Children who were correct on at least four trials on the postswitch block proceeded to the mixed block. The mixed block consisted of 50 trials, including 40 "frequent" and 10 "infrequent" trials presented in a pseudorandom order (with two to five frequent trials preceding each infrequent trial). The frequent dimension corresponded to whichever dimension had been presented in the postswitch block (shape, in this example). For all participants who received the mixed block, however, the trials included in the analyses were truncated after the first 30 mixed-block trials because preliminary analyses indicated possible fatigue effects toward the end of the task, including effects that may interact with age.

The Toolbox DCCS was scored using a newly developed two-vector method that incorporated both accuracy and, for participants who maintained a high level of accuracy (>80% correct), reaction time (RT). On tasks like the DCCS, older children and adults typically slow down (increase in RT) in order to respond accurately. For these participants, RT slowing provides an index of EF "cost." In contrast, younger children (below about 6 years of age) typically fail to show a speed/accuracy trade-off; they continue to respond quickly at the expense of accuracy (Davidson, Amso, Cruess-Anderson, & Diamond, 2006), with the result that only accuracy provides an index of EF cost for these participants.

For all participants, accuracy was considered first and was scored on a scale from 0 to 5. Children were given .125 points (5 points divided by 40 total task trials: 5 pre-, 5 post-, and 30 mixed-block trials) for every correct response they made on trials they received. In other words:

$$\text{Accuracy Score} = 0.125 \times \text{Number Correct Responses} \qquad (1)$$

Performance was scored on the test trials that each participant received, whether these included only the preswitch block, both pre- and postswitch blocks, or all blocks. For children who received only the preswitch block, or only both pre- and postswitch blocks, the final score was equal to the accuracy score. For children who received all blocks, and whose accuracy across all trials was *less* than 80%, the final score was equal to the accuracy score. For participants who received all blocks and whose accuracy was 80% or higher, an RT score was also calculated based on each participant's median RT on correct infrequent trials on the mixed block. Trials with RTs lower than 100 msec or greater than 3 SDs from each participant's mean RT were discarded as outliers prior to calculation of median RT; these trials were unlikely to provide a valid measure of performance.

Like the accuracy score, the RT score ranged from 0 to 5. Because RT tends to have a positively skewed distribution, a log (Base 10) transformation was applied to each participant's median RT score, creating a more normal distribution of scores. Based on the validation data, the minimum RT for scoring was set to 500 msec and the maximum to 3,000 msec. Median RTs that fell outside of this range but within the allowable range of 100–10,000 msec were truncated for the purposes of RT score calculation.[2] That is, RTs between 100 and 500 msec were set equal to 500 msec and RTs between 3,000 msec and 10,000 msec were set equal to 3,000 msec. Scoring of the validation data indicated that this truncation did not introduce any ceiling or floor effects. Log values were algebraically rescaled from a log(500)–log(3,000) range to a 0–5 range. Note that the rescaled scores were reversed such that smaller RT log values are at the upper end of the 0–5 range whereas larger RT log values are at the lower end. Once the rescaled RT scores were obtained, they were added to the accuracy scores for participants who achieved the accuracy criterion of 80% or better.

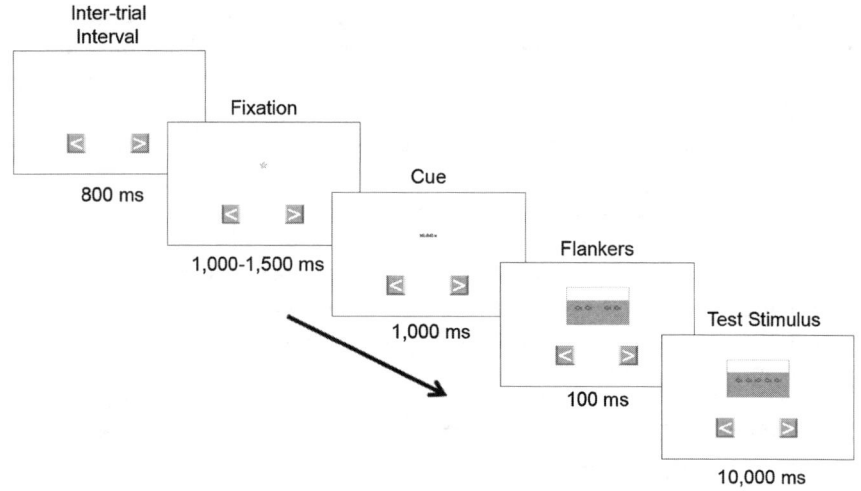

Figure 2.—Trial sequence for the Toolbox Flanker Inhibitory Control and Attention Test (fish block). © 2006–2012 National Institutes of Health and Northwestern University.

Toolbox Flanker Inhibitory Control and Attention Test

The modified version of the flanker task included in the CB consisted of a practice block, a fish block, and an arrows block. In the practice block, which used fish stimuli, children were instructed to press one of two "buttons" on the touch screen corresponding to the direction in which the middle fish was pointing (see Figure 2 for the trial structure and the timing of each stimulus). In order to remind participants to attend to the middle stimulus, the word middle with visually presented to all participants, and also auditorily to those under 12 years of age. As in the Toolbox DCCS, a touch screen monitor was used to record participants' responses, although subsequent research suggests that a simple key press works equally well at all ages.

In the practice block, children were presented with four trials (two congruent and two incongruent) and had to get at least three correct in order to advance to the test trials. If they did not meet this criterion, they received up to three series of four practice trials, and if they still failed to meet criterion, testing was terminated. Seven children failed to meet criterion, and no data were collected from these children. Participants who passed the practice trials then received a block of 25 fish trials, with 16 congruent and 9 incongruent trials presented in pseudorandom order (with 1–3 congruent trials preceding each incongruent trial). Children who got 5 or more of the 9 incongruent trials correct then proceeded to the arrows block. In the arrows block, the stimuli consisted of arrows instead of fish, but the structure of this block was otherwise identical to the fish block (25 trials, with 16 congruent and 9 incongruent).

Scores for the Toolbox Flanker were created using a procedure that was analogous to that used for the Toolbox DCCS, with a two-vector method that incorporated accuracy and, for participants who maintained a high level of accuracy (>80% correct), RT as well. Preliminary analyses again indicated possible fatigue effects in the last few trials of the task, so scoring was based on the first 20 (out of 25) trials in each test block. Accuracy scores and RT scores were calculated using the same formulae that were used for the Toolbox DCCS, and each type of score ranged from 0 to 5. That is, Equation (1) was used to determine accuracy scores (based on both congruent and incongruent trials), and RT data were handled in the same way as in the DCCS. In particular, (a) trials with RTs lower than 100 msec or greater than 3 SDs from each participant's mean RT were discarded as outliers; (b) median RT was calculated based on correct incongruent trials; (c) a log (Base 10) transform was applied to each participant's median RT score; and (d) the minimum RT for scoring was set to 500 msec and the maximum to 3,000 msec, and all allowable scores (range of 100–10,000 msec) outside of this range were reset to the maximum or minimum as appropriate. Once rescaled RT scores (ranging from 0 to 5) were obtained, they were then added to the accuracy scores for participants who achieved the accuracy criterion of 80% or better.

Validation Measures

Convergent Validity Measures

Convergent validity was assessed by examining relations between each new CB measure and existing measures of the same construct. It should be noted, however, that there is often little consensus regarding which measures may be considered established measures of EF in children, and no existing measures can be used across the entire age range of 3–15 years. As a result, different convergent validity measures were used for younger (3–6 years) and older (8–15 years) participants. For both the Toolbox DCCS and the Toolbox Flanker, the Block Design subtest of the Wechsler Preschool and Primary Scale of Intelligence, 3rd Edition (WPPSI–III; Wechsler, 2002) was used for 3 to 6 year olds, and the Delis–Kaplan Executive Function Scales (D-KEFS; Delis, Kaplan, & Kramer, 2001) Color-Word Interference Inhibition raw score was used for 8 to 15 year olds.

The Block Design subtest of the WPPSI–III is a measure of fluid cognition, which is typically highly correlated with EF (e.g., Blair, 2006). In this task, children are shown either a constructed model or a picture of blocks and are asked to recreate the model within a specified time limit using a set of one- or two-color blocks.

The D-KEFS Color-Word test is a Stroop task that provides an index of inhibitory control (or executive attention), and specifically, a measure of the inhibition of an overlearned verbal response in accordance with a set of rules. Participants are timed during three conditions: (1) naming patches of colors; (2) reading basic color words printed in black ink; and (3) naming the color of the ink in which color words are printed. In the last (inhibition) condition, the colors of the ink and the printed color words are incongruent.

Discriminant Validity Measure

The Peabody Picture Vocabulary Test, 4th Edition (PPVT-IV; Dunn & Dunn, 2007) was used as a discriminant measure at all ages. The PPVT-IV is a test of receptive vocabulary and is often used as a proxy for full scale IQ or general developmental level. On each trial, a set of four pictures is provided along with a word describing one of the pictures. The participant is asked to point to or say the number of the picture that best corresponds to the word. The test was administered and scored using the standard protocol. The PPVT-IV was selected in part because it has good psychometric properties within the target age range. In addition, it was attractive as a measure because it could be administered across the entire age range for the battery (ages 3–85 years), allowing for use of the same metric for all ages.

Data Analysis

For the Toolbox DCCS, data from 5 children were judged to be invalid based on the examiner's notes (e.g., child not paying attention, stopping mid task, etc.), 7 children had too few correct trials upon which to base RT scores (i.e., fewer than 2 correct trials), and data from 28 children were excluded from analysis because they were clear outliers for their age (i.e., children 5 years or older who failed to meet the accuracy criterion of 80% correct), leaving a final sample for this measure of $n = 166$. For the Toolbox Flanker inhibitory control measure, data from six children were judged to be invalid based on the examiner's notes, 14 children had too few correct trials upon which to base RT scores (i.e., fewer than 2 correct trials), and data from seven children were excluded from analysis because they were clear outliers for their age (again, based on failing to meet the accuracy criterion), leaving a final sample for this measure of $n = 174$.

For analyses of all NIH Toolbox measures and their corresponding validation measures, normalized scaled scores were created so that all scores would have a common metric with a common distribution, facilitating comparison and interpretation. Normalized scaled scores were created by first ranking the raw scores of all participants between the ages of 3 and 15 years, then applying a normative transformation to the ranks to create a standard normal distribution, and finally rescaling the distribution to have a mean of 10 and a standard deviation of 3. These scaled scores were used in all analyses and not adjusted for age. Intraclass correlation coefficients (*ICC*) with 95% confidence intervals were calculated to evaluate test–retest reliability.

RESULTS

Age Effects

Performance on each NIH Toolbox measure is plotted as a function of age in Figure 3. Correlations between the new NIH Toolbox measures and age are presented in Table 6, shown for the entire sample and for younger (3–6 years) and older (8–15 years) children separately. Across the entire sample, moderate to strong positive correlations were found with age, and for both measures, a cubic model provided the best fit of the data, with $R^2 = .76$ for DCCS and .77 for Flanker. Pairwise comparisons between age groups are reported in Appendix A.

Test–Retest Reliability

ICC are presented in Table 7, as estimates of the test–retest reliability for each new measure. Results indicated that the Toolbox DCCS and Flanker Tests both demonstrate excellent test–retest reliability.

Effects of Repeated Testing

Practice effects were computed as the difference between test and retest normalized scaled scores, with significance of the effect being tested with *t*-tests for dependent means. For the total child group (ages 3–15 years), the

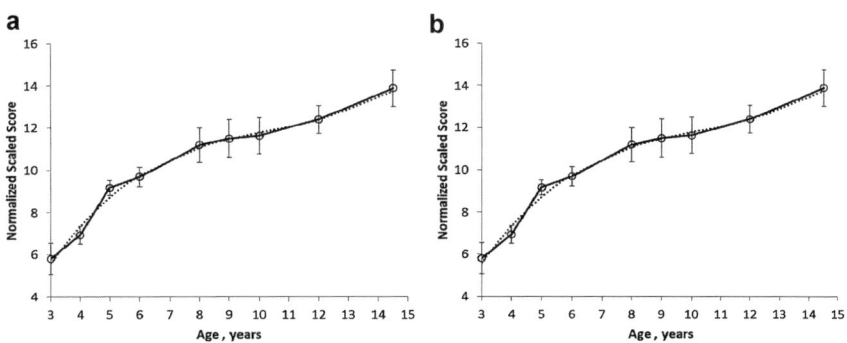

FIGURE 3.—Normalized scaled scores on the Toolbox Dimensional Change Card Sort (DCCS) Test (a) and the Toolbox Flanker Test (b) across age groups. Error bars are ±2 standard errors. Best-fitting polynomial curves are also shown (see text).

TABLE 6

Pearson Correlation Coefficients Between Age and the NIH Toolbox CB Measures of EF and Attention

Sample	Measure	Correlation	n
Whole sample (3–15 years)	Toolbox DCCS	.84**	166
	Toolbox Flanker	.83**	174
Younger group (3–6 years)	Toolbox DCCS	.79**	84
	Toolbox Flanker	.84**	89
Older group (8–15 years)	Toolbox DCCS	.53**	82
	Toolbox Flanker	.44**	85

Note. DCCS = Dimensional Change Card Sort.
**$p < .0001$.© 2006–2012 National Institutes of Health and Northwestern University.

Toolbox DCCS showed no practice effect over an average 2-week test–retest interval: *mean practice effect* = −.04, $SD = 1.20$, $t(47) = -.21$, $p = .83$. The Toolbox Flanker, however, did show a practice effect (*mean* = .51, $SD = 1.14$, $t(48) = 3.15$, $p < .005$).

Construct Validity

Convergent Validity

Correlations were performed between the NIH Toolbox measures and the corresponding convergent validation instruments. Toolbox DCCS scores were positively correlated with WPPSI–III Block Design in 3–6 year olds, $r(74) = .69$, $p < .0001$, and with D-KEFS Inhibition raw scores in children between 8 and 15 years of age, $r(79) = .64$, $p < .0001$. Scores on the Toolbox Flanker were also positively correlated with WPPSI–III Block Design in 3 to 6 year olds, $r(81) = .60$, $p < .0001$, and with D-KEFS Inhibition raw scores in 8–15 year olds, $r(81) = .34$, $p = .002$.

TABLE 7

Test–Retest Intraclass Correlation Coefficients (ICC) for the NIH Toolbox CB Measures of EF and Attention

Measure	ICC	n	95% CI
Toolbox DCCS	.92	48	.86–.95
Toolbox Flanker	.92	49	.86–.95

Note. DCCS, Dimensional Change Card Sort; CI, confidence interval.© 2006–2012 National Institutes of Health and Northwestern University.

Discriminant Validity

High correlations were obtained between the Toolbox measures and PPVT-IV scores, although the magnitude of these correlations declined markedly with age. For younger children (3–6 years), PPVT-IV scores were strongly related to scores on the DCCS, $r(78) = .79$, $p < .0001$, and Flanker, $r(85) = .67$, $p < .0001$). In contrast, for older children (8–15 years), the corresponding correlations were $r(80) = .55$, $p < .0001$ (DCCS), and $r(82) = .44$, $p < .0001$ (Flanker).

Discriminant correlations did not differ significantly from the corresponding convergent correlations.

DISCUSSION

In the current study, we sought to assess the reliability and validity of new measures of EF and attention that are part of the NIH Toolbox CB. New versions of the DCCS and the flanker task were designed to provide assessments of two aspects of EF, cognitive flexibility (Toolbox DCCS) and inhibitory control in the context of visual selective attention (Toolbox Flanker). Together with a separate measure of working memory (see Tulsky et al., Chapter 5, this volume), these measures capture the three aspects of EF identified by Miyake et al. (2000) in their work with adults.

Overall, results reveal excellent developmental sensitivity across childhood, excellent test–retest reliability, and excellent convergent validity (except for the Toolbox Flanker, which showed adequate convergent validity among 8–15 year olds). Correlations between the new NIH Toolbox measures and corresponding convergent measures were generally quite high, although for younger children, they were higher for the DCCS than for the flanker measures.

Historically, it has been difficult to study developmental changes from early childhood through adolescence due to the lack of measures that can be used across the entire age range. The lack of common measures has made it impossible to separate differences in task demands at different ages from genuine developmental changes. The new measures were designed to address this difficulty, and several important developmental trends were noted in the data reported here. First, correlations between the new NIH Toolbox measures and age were higher for younger children (3–6 years) than for older children (8–15 years). This pattern may be consistent with Best and Miller's (2010) suggestion that early age-related changes in EF result from fundamental changes to the structure of cognition (e.g., the emergence of higher order rule use; see Zelazo et al., 2003) whereas improvements in EF occurring in early and middle adolescence are a function of ongoing refinement of those cognitive skills as a function of experience and opportunity.

Perhaps the most interesting developmental trend to emerge from the data, however, was the finding that correlations between the NIH Toolbox measures and receptive vocabulary declined with age, dropping by 43% for the Toolbox DCCS and 24% for the Toolbox Flanker. This finding suggests that as children develop, EF becomes increasingly differentiated from receptive vocabulary ability, which was used as a proxy for general intellectual level. Additional research using the CB is currently underway as part of the norming process (see Bauer & Zelazo, Chapter 9, this volume), and the results from this much larger study will be better able to address age-related changes in the interrelations among cognitive domains. In any case, however, the current findings support the suggestion that key aspects of neurocognitive development involve the experience-dependent functional specialization of neural networks. A classic example of this process occurs in perceptual development. Initially, for example, occipital cortical areas involved in vision are activated by cross modal input from other sensory modalities (see Collignon, Voss, Lassonde, & Lepore, 2009; Spector & Maurer, 2009). With normal visual experience, however, visual inputs to occipital cortex are reinforced whereas cross modal inputs from other perceptual systems are eliminated and/or inhibited. A similar process may occur more broadly in brain development, including in higher-order association areas (such as prefrontal cortex) that integrate information from lower-order, earlier developing areas such as visual cortex.

Having methodologically sound measurement tools that can be used over a broad age span will be of considerable value to the field for a number of reasons, from basic scientific to applied. On the basic side, the CB will greatly facilitate the description of cognitive development, helping us to map development with greater precision and in more detail, and to follow a much wider range of developmental pathways longitudinally. On the more applied side, this advance in descriptive power will be very useful for intervention studies, and it will immediately provide opportunities to identify key mechanisms underlying important developmental outcomes, including academic and social success.

EF and attention have emerged as major foci of research in part because they predict a wide range of important developmental outcomes. Indeed, numerous developmental disorders are characterized by deficits in EF, which suggests that its development is fragile and easily disrupted. At the same time, however, there is growing evidence that EF and attention are malleable—perhaps especially during the preschool years, a period of substantial change in EF, attention, and prefrontal cortex, that occurs just prior to a marked increase in the extent to which self-regulation is required of children (e.g., as they transition to school). The far-reaching consequences of EF and attention underscore the importance of a complete understanding of their developmental course, and the NIH Toolbox CB represents an important step toward achieving this goal.

REFERENCES

Beck, D. M., Schaefer, C., Pang, K., & Carlson, S. M. (2011). Executive function in preschool children: Test–retest reliability. *Journal of Cognition and Development*, **12**, 169–193.

Best, J. R., & Miller, P. H. (2010). A developmental perspective on executive function. *Child Development*, **81**, 1641–1660.

Blair, C. (2006). How similar are fluid cognition and general intelligence? A developmental neuroscience perspective on fluid cognition as an aspect of human cognitive ability. *Behavioral and Brain Sciences*, **29**, 109–125.

Blair, C., & Razza, R. A. (2007). Relating effortful control, executive function, and false belief understanding to emerging math and literacy ability in kindergarten. *Child Development*, **78**, 647–663.

Carlson, S. M., Davis, A. C., & Leach, J. G. (2005). Less is more: Executive function and symbolic representation in preschool children. *Psychological Science*, **16**, 609–616.

Collignon, O., Voss, P., Lassonde, M., & Lepore, F. (2009). Cross-modal plasticity for the spatial processing of sounds in visually deprived subjects. *Experimental Brain Research*, **192**, 343–358.

Davidson, M. C., Amso, D., Cruess-Anderson, L., & Diamond, A. (2006). Development of cognitive control and executive functions from 4–13 years: Evidence from manipulations of memory, inhibition and task switching. *Neuropsychologia*, **44**, 2037–2078.

Delis, D. C., Kaplan, E., & Kramer, J. H. (2001). *Delis–Kaplan executive function system.* San Antonio, TX: Pearson (The Psychological Corporation).

Diamond, A., Barnett, W. S., Thomas, J., & Munro, S. (2007). Preschool program improves cognitive control. *Science*, **318**, 1387–1388.

Diamond, A., & Kirkham, N. (2005). Not quite as grown-up as we like to think. *Psychological Science*, **16**, 291–297.

Dick, A. S., Overton, W. F., & Kovacs, S. L. (2005). The development of symbolic coordination: Representation of imagined objects, executive function, and theory of mind. *Journal of Cognition and Development*, **6**, 133–161.

Dunn, L. M., & Dunn, D. M. (2007). *Peabody picture vocabulary test* (4th ed.). San Antonio, TX: Pearson.

Eigsti, I. M., Zayas, V., Mischel, W., Shoda, Y., Ayduk, O., Dadlani, M, et al. (2006). Predicting cognitive control from preschool to late adolescence and young adulthood. *Psychological Science*, **17**, 478–484.

Eriksen, B. A., & Eriksen, C. W. (1974). Effects of noise letters upon the identification of a target letter in a nonsearch task. *Perception and Psychophysics*, **16**, 143–149.

Fan, J., McCandliss, B. D., Sommer, T., Raz, A., & Posner, M. I. (2002). Testing the efficiency and independence of attentional networks. *Journal of Cognitive Neuroscience*, **14**, 340–347.

Frye, D., Zelazo, P. D., & Palfai, T. (1995). Theory of mind and rule-based reasoning. *Cognitive Development*, **10**, 483–527.

Grant, D. A., & Berg, E. A. (1948). A behavioral analysis of degree of reinforcement and ease of shifting to new responses in a Weigl-type-card-sorting problem. *Journal of Experimental Psychology*, **38**, 404–411.

Hirschfeld, L. A., & Gelman, S. (1994). *Mapping the mind: Domain specificity in cognition and culture*. New York: Cambridge University Press.

Johnson, M. H., & Munakata, Y. (2005). Processes of change in brain and cognitive development. *Trends in Cognitive Sciences*, **9**(3), 152–158.

Kirkham, N., Cruess, L. M., & Diamond, A. (2003). Helping children apply their knowledge to their behavior on a dimension-switching task. *Developmental Science*, **6**, 449–467.

Lehto, J. E., Juujärvi, P., Kooistra, L., & Pulkkinen, L. (2003). Dimensions of executive functioning: Evidence from children. *British Journal of Developmental Psychology*, **21**, 59–80.

McAuley, T., & White, D. A. (2011). A latent variables examination of processing speed, response inhibition, and working memory during typical development. *Journal of Experimental Child Psychology*, **108**, 453–468.

McClelland, M. M., Cameron, C. E., Connor, C. M., Farris, C. L., Jewkes, A. M., & Morrison, F. J. (2007). Links between behavioral regulation and preschoolers' literacy, vocabulary, and math skills. *Developmental Psychology*, **43**, 947–959.

Miyake, A., Friedman, N. P., Emerson, M. J., Witzki, A. H., Howerter, A., & Wager, T. D. (2000). The unity and diversity of executive functions and their contributions to complex "frontal lobe" tasks: A latent variable analysis. *Cognitive Psychology*, **41**, 49–100.

Moffit, T. E., Arsenault, L., Belsky, D., Dickson, N., Hancox, R. J., Harrington, H, et al. (2011). A gradient of childhood self-control predicts health, wealth, and public safety. *Proceedings of the National Academy of Sciences United States of America*, **108**, 2693–2698.

Moriguchi, Y., & Hiraki, K. (2009). Neural origin of cognitive shifting in young children. *Proceedings of the National Academy of Sciences United States of America*, **106**, 6017–6021.

Morton, J. B., Bosma, R., & Ansari, D. (2009). Age-related changes in brain activation associated with dimension shifts of attention: An fMRI study. *NeuroImage*, **46**, 249–256.

Posner, M. I., & Boies, S. J. (1971). Components of attention. *Psychological Review*, **78**, 391–408.

Raz, A., & Buhle, J. (2006). Typologies of attentional networks. *Nature Reviews Neuroscience*, **7**, 367–379.

Riggs, N. R., Greenberg, M. T., Kusche, C. A., & Pentz, M. A. (2006). The mediational role of neurocognition in the behavioral outcomes of a social-emotional prevention program in elementary school students: Effects of the PATHS curriculum. *Prevention Science*, **7**, 91–102.

Roberts, M. J. (2007). *Integrating the mind: Domain general versus domain specific processes in higher cognition*. New York: Psychology Press.

Rueda, M. R., Fan, J., McCandliss, B. D., Halparin, J. D., Gruber, D. B., Lercari, L. P., et al. (2004). Development of attentional networks in childhood. *Neuropsychologia*, **42**, 1029–1040.

Rueda, M. R., Posner, M. I., & Rothbart, M. K. (2005). The development of executive function: Contributions to the emergence of self-regulation. *Developmental Neuropsychology*, **28**, 573–594.

Spector, F., & Maurer, D. (2009). Synesthesia: A new approach to understanding the development of perception. *Developmental Psychology*, **45**, 175–189.

Stroop, J. R. (1935). Studies of interference in serial verbal reactions. *Journal of Experimental Psychology*, **18**, 643–662.

Visu-Petra, L., Benga, O., Tincas, I., & Miclea, M. (2007). Visual-spatial processing in children and adolescents with Down's syndrome: A computerized assessment of memory skills. *Journal of Intellectual Disability Research*, **51**, 942–952.

Wechsler, D. (2002). *Wechsler Preschool and Primary Scale of Intelligence* (3rd ed.). San Antonio, TX: Pearson.

Wiebe, S. A., Espy, K. A., & Charak, D. (2008). Using confirmatory factor analysis to understand executive control in preschool children: I. Latent structure. *Developmental Psychology*, **44**, 575–587.

Wiebe, S. A., Sheffield, T., Nelson, J. M., Clark, C. A. C., Chevalier, N., & Espy, K. (2011). The structure of executive function in 3-year-olds. *Journal of Experimental Child Psychology*, **108**, 436–452.

Zelazo, P. D. (2006). The Dimensional Change Card Sort: A method of assessing executive function in children. *Nature Protocols*, **1**, 297–301.

Zelazo, P. D., Carlson, S. M., & Kesek, A., (2008) Development of executive function in childhood. In C. A. Nelson, & M. Luciana (Eds.) *Handbook of developmental cognitive neuroscience* (2nd. ed., pp. 553–574). Cambridge, MA: MIT Press.

Zelazo, P. D., Craik, F. I. M., & Booth, L. (2004). Executive function across the life span. *Acta Psychologica*, **115**, 167–184.

Zelazo, P. D., Müller, U., Frye, D., & Marcovitch, S. (2003). The development of executive function in early childhood. *Monographs of the Society for Research in Child Development*, **68**(3), Serial No. 274.

NOTE

2. One participant had median RTs >3,000 msec on both the DCCS and the Flanker (see below). For each test, there were three additional participants who had median RT >3,000 msec.

III. NIH TOOLBOX COGNITION BATTERY (CB): MEASURING EPISODIC MEMORY

Patricia J. Bauer, Sureyya S. Dikmen, Robert K. Heaton, Dan Mungas, Jerry Slotkin, and Jennifer L. Beaumont

ABSTRACT One of the most significant domains of cognition is episodic memory, which allows for rapid acquisition and long-term storage of new information. For purposes of the NIH Toolbox, we devised a new test of episodic memory. The nonverbal NIH Toolbox Picture Sequence Memory Test (TPSMT) requires participants to reproduce the order of an arbitrarily ordered sequence of pictures presented on a computer. To adjust for ability, sequence length varies from 6 to 15 pictures. Multiple trials are administered to increase reliability. Pediatric data from the validation study revealed the TPSMT to be sensitive to age-related changes. The task also has high test–retest reliability and promising construct validity. Steps to further increase the sensitivity of the instrument to individual and age-related variability are described.

In this chapter, we introduce the NIH Toolbox Picture Sequence Memory Test (TPSMT), a measure developed as a test of episodic memory for ages 3–85 years. Episodic memory permits rapid learning and retention of new information. It is the basis for formation of memories of the mundane—such as where the car was parked last—to the special events that constitute one's life story or personal past.

Subdomain Definition

Evidence from nonhuman animals, patient populations, and typically developing children and adults makes clear that memory is not a unitary construct. Rather, it is comprised of different systems of information encoding, storage, and retrieval. One major distinction is the dichotomy between maintenance of information over the short term, and over the long term

---

Corresponding author: Patricia J. Bauer, Department of Psychology, Emory University, 36 Eagle Row, Atlanta, GA 30322, email: patricia.bauer@emory.edu

(long-term memory). Short-term or working memory is discussed in Tulsky and colleagues (Chapter 5, this volume); long-term memory is the subject of the current chapter. Within long-term memory there is a distinction between procedural (or implicit, or nondeclarative) memory and declarative (or explicit) memory (e.g., Squire, Knowlton, & Musen, 1993; Tulving, 2000). Procedural, implicit, or nondeclarative memories guide behavior but seemingly require no effort to retrieve and are not accessible to consciousness. Work with animal models and human patients makes clear that the procedural memory system remains relatively intact in aging and is virtually unaffected by neurological conditions and diseases that target the medial temporal lobe structures involved in the declarative memory system (Churchill, Stanis, Press, Kushelev, & Greenough, 2003; Reber, Martinez, & Weintraub, 2003).

In contrast to procedural memory, declarative or explicit memory is effortful and involves conscious recollection of information that is potentially verbally accessible. The declarative memory system is further divided into semantic and episodic memory (e.g., Squire, 2004). Semantic memory is specialized for storage of timeless, placeless facts, concepts, and the vocabulary to describe them. Knowledge stored in semantic memory typically is long lasting, which is the basis for reference to semantic memory as "crystallized intelligence." Semantic memory is resistant to decline with age and to neurological insult. The construct of semantic memory is measured by the Toolbox Picture Vocabulary Test and the Toolbox Oral Reading Recognition Test (see Gershon et al., Chapter 4, this volume). In contrast, episodic memory is specialized for storage of unique events or experiences encoded in a time-specific manner. Episodic memory is fragile and time-limited (though some memories, such as those of special, personally relevant events, may endure over long periods of time), and it is sensitive to decay and interference, as well as to both normal aging and many brain diseases.

Importance During Childhood

Episodic memory allows for rapid, even one-trial, learning of new information and for retention of information for later retrieval. As such, it provides the building blocks for cognitive growth during development and throughout the lifespan. Its importance to mental life is nowhere more in evidence than in the historic case of the patient HM, who as a result of surgery to the medial–temporal lobe, lost the capacity for forming new episodic memories (e.g., Corkin, 2002). As well, the relatively protracted course of development of episodic memory is a major source of one of the most robust phenomena in the memory literature, namely, infantile or childhood amnesia: the relative paucity among adults of memories of unique events for the first 3–4 years of life (see Bauer, 2007, for a review). Thus, this cognitive ability is critical for achieving a concept of self that is continuous over time, for independence, education, and success in personal and professional activities of daily life throughout the lifespan. The centrality of episodic memory explains why it is the most frequently measured form of memory and why it is included in the CB.

The course of development of episodic memory is protracted, with pronounced changes throughout the first two decades of life (see Bauer, 2007; Bauer, Larkina, & Deocampo, 2011, for reviews). In infancy, the ability is measured using nonverbal tasks, such as elicited and deferred imitation (props are used to produce a specific action or sequence of actions that the infant is permitted to imitate either immediately, after a delay, or both; e.g., Bauer & Shore, 1987; Bauer & Mandler, 1989). Use of imitation-based tasks in the first 3 years of life has revealed age-related increases in the length of time over which memory is preserved, in the robustness of memory, and in the reliability with which it is observed (e.g., Bauer, Wenner, Dropik, & Wewerka, 2000). Developmental changes are especially apparent in the ability to remember the temporal order of events (e.g., Bauer et al., 2000), making this aspect of episodic memory a target for the CB.

Episodic memory continues to develop throughout childhood and into adolescence. There are age-related increases in the amount of information that children remember. For example, relative to younger children, older children remember longer lists of items (see, e.g., Bjorklund, Dukes, & Brown, 2009, for a review), thus making list length a prime target for exploitation in tests of episodic memory designed for wide age ranges (see below). With development, children's memory becomes more deliberate and strategic, with resulting increases in the organization that children impose on to-be-remembered material (e.g., Bjorklund et al., 2009). In addition, children become more aware of their own and others' memory processes (i.e., increases in metamemory), enabling them to recruit information-processing resources in the service of increased memory demands. As a result, we may expect to see age-related increases in the amount of information children are able to remember, and in their ability to bring organization to it.

The overall importance of episodic memory to typical development is brought into stark relief in pediatric populations in whom the function is impaired. The most striking example is a population who as infants and very young children, sustained damage to the medial–temporal lobe structures that support declarative memory (see below). Without exception, individuals in this population of so-called *developmental amnesics* experienced difficulty learning in school and deficits on episodic memory tasks (Gadian et al., 2000). Importantly, the damage sustained by this population is confined to the neural structures involved in declarative memory in general and episodic memory in particular, described next.

Relations of Domain With Brain Function

Encoding, storage, and retrieval of episodic memories depend on a multi-component network involving the temporal lobe (including hippocampus and surrounding cortices) and other cortical area (including prefrontal cortex and limbic/temporal association areas) (e.g., Eichenbaum & Cohen, 2001; Zola & Squire, 2000). Specifically, the process of encoding of new memories begins as the elements that constitute an event register across primary sensory areas (auditory, somatosensory, visual). Inputs from the primary cortices are projected to unimodal association areas, where they are integrated into whole percepts of what objects sound, feel, and look like. Unimodal association areas in turn project to polymodal prefrontal, posterior, and limbic association cortices where inputs from the different sense modalities are integrated and maintained over brief delays (seconds; e.g., Petrides, 1995). For maintenance beyond the short term, the inputs must be stabilized or consolidated, a task attributed to medial temporal structures, in concert with cortical areas (McGaugh, 2000). Eventually, new traces become stabilized, permitting long-term storage in the neocortex. The prefrontal cortex is implicated in memory retrieval (e.g., Cabeza et al., 2004; Maguire, 2001). Demands on the temporal–cortical network are especially high when tasks require free recall versus recognition, and memory for temporal order information versus for items alone (e.g., Shimamura, Janowsky, & Squire, 1990). As discussed earlier, these conditions are those under which the most pronounced age-related differences are observed, thus informing design of the Toolbox measure for episodic memory.

Each of the brain regions involved in episodic memory, as well as the connections between them, undergoes substantial postnatal developmental change that extends well into the second decade of life (see Bauer, 2008, for a review). Throughout childhood and into adolescence there are gradual increases in hippocampal volume (e.g., Gogtay et al., 2004; Pfluger et al., 1999; Utsunomiya, Takano, Okazaki, & Mistudome, 1999) and in myelination in the hippocampal region (Arnold & Trojanowski, 1996; Benes, Turtle, Khan, & Farol, 1994; Schneider, Il'yasov, Hennig, & Martin, 2004). In the prefrontal cortex, pruning of synapses to adult levels does not begin until late childhood; adult levels are not reached until late adolescence or even early adulthood (Huttenlocher, 1979; Huttenlocher & Dabholkar, 1997). Although there are well-documented reciprocal connections between the hippocampus and frontal lobes, their development has not been fully elucidated (see Barbas, 2000; Fuster, 2002). Finally, it is not until adolescence that neurotransmitters such as acetylcholine reach adult levels (Benes, 2001).

Developmental changes in the neural structures and network that support episodic memory may be expected to have functional consequences. Consistent with this expectation, Sowell, Delis, Stiles, and Jernigan (2001) reported relations between structural changes in the medial–temporal and frontal regions, as measured by MRI, and performance on behavioral tests of memory. Children with structurally more mature medial–temporal lobe regions performed at higher levels on spatial memory tasks. Children with structurally more mature frontal cortices performed at higher levels on verbal and spatial memory tasks. Increases in myelination also are correlated with functional changes (Olesen, Nagy, Westerberg, & Klingberg, 2003). Developmental studies of the magnitude and patterns of neural activation during episodic memory task performance are rare and have focused on encoding only. Ofen et al. (2007) found that in regions of prefrontal cortex associated with successful encoding, activations increased with age. Although medial–temporal activations were associated with successful encoding, they were not age-related (although see Menon, Boyett-Anderson, & Reiss, 2005).

Among children with known compromise of the medial–temporal structures, there are clear deficits on episodic memory tasks. For example, infants born with low iron stores as a result of failed regulation of maternal glucose during pregnancy (i.e., poorly controlled maternal gestational diabetes) show impaired performance on imitation-based tests of episodic memory from infancy through the preschool years (e.g., DeBoer, Wewerka, Bauer, Georgieff, & Nelson, 2005; Riggins, Miller, Bauer, Georgieff, & Nelson, 2009). Individuals with developmental amnesia provide another example: When tested as adolescents or adults, they show impaired performance on standard tests of episodic memory as well as age-appropriate analogues of imitation-based tasks (Adlam, Vargha-Khadem, Mishkin, & de Haan, 2005). In summary, the neural substrate that supports episodic memory is relatively well understood. Compromised development in the implicated structures, especially in the medial–temporal components of the network, is associated with impaired performance.

Toolbox Picture Sequence Memory Test

To measure episodic memory as part of the CB, we developed a new measure, the NIH TPSMT. The measure is derived from imitation-based tasks (elicited and deferred imitation) developed by Bauer and her colleagues for research with pre- and early-verbal infants and young children (e.g., see Bauer, 2005, 2006, 2007, for descriptions and discussion). For infant and young child populations, the stimuli are three-dimensional props used to produce sequences of action that the infant or child imitates. For the CB, the stimuli are sequences of pictured objects and activities presented on a computer screen.

The TPSMT developed for the CB addresses several needs. First, it provides a measure of episodic memory for children below 5 years of age. Based on the success of imitation-based measures even in infancy, the decision was made to adjust the procedure upward to cover the full age range (3–85 years). Development of the NIH TPSMT also addresses a need for tests that can be readily used with nonEnglish speakers. Finally, multiple alternate forms of the TPSMT can easily be created to reduce practice effects in longitudinal studies. In the validation study described in this chapter, three alternate forms were included. Total administration time is approximately 10 min. The validation study included the full age range of the NIH Toolbox, ages 3–85 years.

METHOD

Participants

The participants in the validation study are described in detail in Weintraub et al. (Chapter 1, this volume; Table 2).

Measure Development

The task stimuli for the NIH TPSMT are sequences of pictured objects and activities presented on a computer screen (see Figure 4). The objects and activities are thematically related but with no inherent order. The general themes are "Working on the farm," "Playing at the park," and "Going to the fair." Although there are no inherent constraints on the order in which the activities in the sequences must occur, the pictures are presented in a specific order that the participant must remember and then reproduce. This requirement is made clear in verbal instructions as well as through practice sequences (see below). The level of difficulty of the task for different age ranges was determined during pilot testing. The number of pictures the participants were required to order ranged from 6-picture sequences to 15-picture sequences.

For the test itself, color-illustrated pictures appear one at a time on the computer monitor in a fixed order. Each picture originally is displayed in the

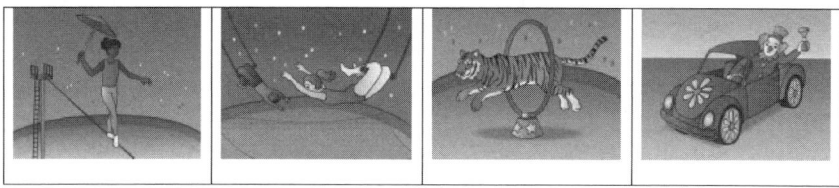

FIGURE 4.—Four-step practice sequence with "circus" theme: Walk a tightrope, swing on the trapeze, jump through the hoop, and drive the funny car.
© 2006–2012 National Institutes of Health and Northwestern University.

center of the computer screen, as a 3″ × 5″ image. As it appears, a recording briefly describes the content of each picture. The duration of presentation for each picture is 2.2 sec. Once described, the picture reduces in size and is translocated to its position in the sequence (requiring 1.5 sec), making way for the next picture, until all pictures in a sequence have been displayed. After 3 sec during which the entire sequence is shown, the pictures are placed in a random spatial array at the center of the screen. For the validation study described in this report, participants used a touch screen to "move" each picture to its correct location in the sequence. Participants were permitted as much time as necessary to complete their responses. Three trials were administered to improve test score variability and test–retest reliability (Strauss, Sherman, & Spreen, 2006); the same sequence was presented on each trial.

For all ages, practice sequences are administered prior to administration of the first test trial to orient participants to the TPSMT task and to provide experience moving the pictures to the correct position in the sequence. For the validation study, for young children, the first practice sequence involved 3 pictures that followed a logical order. Specifically, the sequence involved putting a cake into an oven, frosting it, and then putting candles on the cake. The logical sequence of pictures was intended to reinforce for children the importance of placing the pictures in the correct temporal order. After the pictures in the practice sequence were displayed, children were given practice ordering the pictures. Errors were corrected. After successful completion of the first practice sequence, children were administered two additional practice trials that were 3 and 4 pictures in length, respectively. The 3- and 4-picture sequences had no inherent constraints on their order. Participants ages 5 years and older received one 3-picture and one 4-picture practice sequence; none of their practice sequences had inherent constraints on their order.

Based on pilot testing the following sequence lengths were administered to the different age groups: For ages 3–4 years: 6 pictures; 5–6 years: 9 pictures; 8 years: 12 pictures; 9–60 years: 15 pictures, 65–85 years: 9 pictures. In the next phase of measure development, we will test possible means of adjusting sequence length on-line, in response to participants' performance (see Discussion Section).

Scoring

The participant's score on the TPSMT is derived from the cumulative number of adjacent pairs of pictures remembered correctly over three learning trials. Adjacent pairs are two adjacent pictures placed in consecutive, ascending order. Thus, pictures placed in the orders 1–2 and 2–3 would receive credit, whereas pictures placed in the orders 1–3 and 3–15 would not receive credit (because they are not consecutive). For example, for a 6-picture sequence, the sequence of placement 1–2–3–5–4–6, would result in a score of

2: one point would be awarded for each of the adjacent pairs 1–2 and 2–3. No points would be earned for the correctly ordered pairs 3–5 and 4–6 because they items are nonadjacent. For each trial, the possible number of adjacent pairs is the number of pictures in the sequence, −1. The total possible number of adjacent pairs is the sum of the adjacent-pairs scores across trials.

Validation Measures

Convergent validity was assessed with correlations between TPSMT and established measures of memory. Evidence of discriminant validity was tested with correlations with a validation measure of a *different* cognitive construct, namely vocabulary. We expected the correlations with other memory measures to be high and with vocabulary to be lower.

Convergent Validity

One impetus for development of the TPSMT was that there did not exist a single measure that could be used across the age span of 3–85 years. In fact, neither was there a single measure that could be used within the target age span of 3–15 years. As a result, for purposes of examination of convergent validity, different validation measures were used for ages 3–6 years and ages 8–15 years. For children 3–6 years of age, we selected the sentence repetition subtest of the Developmental Neuropsychological Assessment, 2nd Edition (NEPSY-II; Korkman, Kirk, & Kemp, 2007). The NEPSY-II Sentence Repetition subtest involves an examiner reading a series of sentences of increasing complexity and length. The participant is required to recall each sentence after it is presented. The measure was selected because of its good psychometric properties within the target age range and because it is relatively brief to administer. The subtest was administered and scored using the standard protocol. For analysis we used the Sentence Repetition Total Score.

For children 8–15 years, two different measures were used, one using verbal and the other visuospatial information: the Rey Auditory Verbal Learning Test (RAVLT) and the Brief Visuospatial Memory Test-Revised (BVMT-R; Benedict, 1997). These measures were selected because they have good psychometric properties within the target age range and combined, they sample multiple modalities of learning. In the RAVLT, an examiner reads aloud a list of 15 words, at the rate of one word per second. The test-taker's task is to repeat as many words as possible, in any order. The test was administered and scored using the standard protocol, with the exception that only three trials, rather than five, were administered. In analysis, we used the total score of the three learning trials. The BVMT-R is designed to measure visuospatial memory. The examinee views six geometric figures on a page after which the figures are removed from view. The examinee then is asked to draw as many of the figures as possible from memory in their correct location.

The test was administered and scored using the standard protocol. The score used in analysis was the total score of the three learning trials. Scores on the RAVLT and BVMT-R were strongly correlated with one another, $r(n = 83) = .35, p < .001$. Therefore, to simplify data analysis, for the 8 to 15 year olds, we created a combined validation memory score, which was the mean of performance on the two separate measures.

Discriminant Validity Measure

The Peabody Picture Vocabulary Test, 4th Edition (PPVT-IV; Dunn & Dunn, 2007) was used as a discriminant measure at all ages. The PPVT-IV is a test of receptive vocabulary and is often used as a proxy for full scale IQ or general developmental level. On each trial, a set of 4 pictures is provided along with a word describing one of the pictures. The examinee is asked to point to or say the number of the picture that best corresponds to the word. The test was administered and scored using the standard protocol. The PPVT-IV was selected in part because it has good psychometric properties within the target age range. In addition, it was attractive as a measure because it could be administered across the entire age range for the battery (ages 3–85 years), allowing for use of the same metric for all ages.

Data Analysis

As described in Zelazo et al. (Chapter 2, this volume), normalized scaled scores were used for all analyses. Pearson correlation coefficients between age and test performance were calculated to assess the ability of the TPSMT for detecting developmental growth during childhood. Intraclass correlation coefficients (*ICC*) with 95% confidence intervals were calculated to evaluate test–retest reliability. Convergent validity was assessed with correlations between the TPSMT and the NEPSY-II (ages 3–6 years), and the TPSMT and the mean of the RAVLT and BVMT-R (8–15 years); discriminant validity was assessed with correlations between the TPSMT and PPVT-IV scores (all ages).

RESULTS

Age Effects

The NIH TPSMT provides a valid test of age-related differences in learning and episodic memory, as evidenced by strong associations between the TPSMT and age. As depicted in Figure 5, scores on the TPSMT increased with age. Pairwise comparisons between age groups are reported in Appendix A. Across the 3- to 15-year age span, the correlation with age was $r(202) = .78$, $p < .001$. A quadratic model provided the best fit of the data, with $R^2 = .70$. For the 3- to 6-year age group, the correlation was $r(115) = .69, p < .001$;

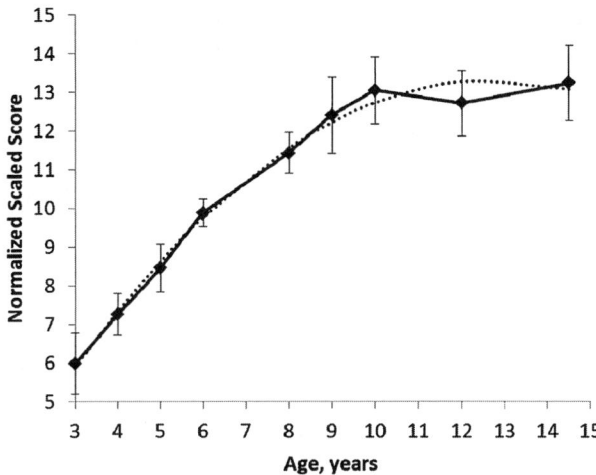

Figure 5.—Normalized scaled scores on the Toolbox Picture Sequence Memory Test across age groups. Error bars are ±2 standard errors. Best-fitting polynomial curve is also shown (see text).

within this group, the correlation between age and performance on the sentence repetition subtest of the NEPSY-II was .58. Thus, the TPSMT proved a nominally stronger relation with age than the validation measure. For the 8- to 15-year age group, the correlation with age was $r(85) = .26$, $p = .016$. Within this group, the correlation between age and performance on the average validation measure was $r(85) = .44$, $p < .001$. Thus, for the 8–15 year olds, relative to the validation measure, the TPSMT was not as sensitive to age-related improvements in performance.

Test–Retest Reliability

The test–retest reliability of the TPSMT was excellent in the full sample of children age 3–15 years, as evidenced by a high intraclass correlation: $ICC = .76$ (95% confidence interval: .64–.85; $n = 66$).

Effect of Repeated Testing

Practice effects were computed as the difference between test and retest normalized scaled scores, with significance of the effect being tested with t tests for dependent means. For the total child group (ages 3–15 years, $n = 66$), the TPSMT showed a practice effect over an average 2-week test–retest interval: *mean practice effect* $= .99$, $SD = 1.88$, $t(65) = 4.27$, $p < .0001$.

Construct Validity

Convergent Validity

For children 3–6 years of age, the TPSMT was moderately correlated with the Sentence Repetition subtest of the NEPSY-II (the validation measure): $r(110) = .50$, $p < .001$. For children 8–15 years of age, the TPSMT was moderately correlated with the mean of the two gold-standard measures of memory (RAVLT and BVMT-R): $r(84) = .47$, $p < .001$. These correlations provide evidence of adequate convergent validity.

Discriminant Validity

For children 3–6 years of age, the correlation between the TPSMT and the PPVT-IV was higher than expected: $r(112) = .58$, $p < .001$, and nominally higher than the correlation with the convergent validity measure. However, the validation NEPSY-II scores also were correlated with PPVT-IV scores: $r(109) = .67$, $p < .001$. Thus, the problem with discriminant validity does not appear to be unique to the TPSMT in the young age group. In the older age group, the correlation between the TPSMT and the PPVT-IV was low, as expected: $r(84) = .28$, $p = .009$.

Discriminant correlations did not differ significantly from the corresponding convergent correlations.

DISCUSSION

The NIH TPSMT is a new measure of learning and episodic memory developed for use across the age span of 3–85 years. It is based on the nonverbal elicited or deferred imitation task designed for use with preverbal infants and early-verbal children. The TPSMT proved to be a valid assessment of age-related changes in episodic learning and memory, as indexed by a strong correlation with age. In spite of the potential for artifactual relations with age as a result of the confound between age and sequence length, the pattern of performance was consistent with true age effects. That is, because sequence length increased with age, the maximum number of correctly ordered adjacent pairs that the children could receive also increased with age: 3 and 4 year olds were tested on sequence length 6; 5 and 6 year olds were tested on sequence length 9; 8 year olds were tested on sequence length 12; and 9–15 year olds were tested on sequence length 15. As a result, the maximum scores that children could earn over three trials were 15, 24, 33, and 48, respectively. Examination of Figure 5 shows that TPSMT scores increased in a linear fashion from age 3 to 9 years, without evidence of departures from linearity at ages where the sequence length changed (e.g., age 4 years vs. age 5 years). This is supportive of a true age effect. Examination of effect sizes between age groups (available from the authors) also was consistent with a true age effect.

The TPSMT also showed strong test/retest reliability within the sample of children ages 3–15 ($ICC = .76$). The assessment of convergent and discriminant validity also was quite promising, with one notable exception involving the younger age group. For the older age group of 8–15 years, the correlation of the TPSMT with the combined validation measure of memory was moderate and higher than the correlation with the measure of vocabulary, as expected. For the younger age group, however, the TPSMT correlated equally highly with the validation measures of memory and also of vocabulary. The lack of discriminant validity was not a problem unique to the TPSMT, however: the validation measure of memory (Sentence Repetition of the NEPSY-II) was even more strongly correlated with the vocabulary test (i.e., the PPVT-IV) than was the TPSMT. As discussed in more detail in Mungus et al. (Chapter 7, this volume), there is evidence of the gradual differentiation of cognitive skills over the course of development, and it is difficult to detect variance associated with any single domain of function within the 3- to 6-year age range.

The NIH TPSMT shows substantial promise as a means of assessment of learning and episodic memory within the 3- to 15-year age range; as described in Weintraub et al. (2013), it also shows promise for young to older adults. Norming will provide a substantial, empirical resource for normative expectations for performance at different ages and for different demographically defined groups. Several changes will be made to the instrument in the norming phase. First, rather than using a touch-screen, participants will register their responses on the TPSMT using a mouse. The change in administration will be made to lessen the demand for specialized equipment for the CB. Participants who are uncomfortable using a mouse will be encouraged to point to the screen and the test administrator will operate the mouse. As such, the change is expected to have a negligible impact on performance. Second, in an effort to avoid floor effects, the norming study will feature different practice trials that are expected to more effectively convey task requirements. This change is expected to aid the youngest children and the elderly, in particular. Third, also in an effort to further improve the sensitivity of the instrument—this time to avoid ceiling effects—18-step sequences have been developed for potential use with participants who achieve perfect or near-perfect performance on shorter sequence lengths. In the norming study, some participants 8–60 years of age will be tested on a 15-step sequence on Trial 1 and 18-step sequences on Trials 2 and 3, whereas others will experience 15-step sequences on each test trial (the procedure followed in the present research). A similar scheme will be implemented for the shorter sequence lengths as well (for participants younger than 8 years and older than 60 years). The resulting data will be used to create item response functions and to explore the feasibility of computerized adaptive testing (CAT) that would permit selection of sequence length based on a participant's own performance.

In conclusion, NIH TPSMT is a newly developed measure of episodic memory for use across the 3- to 85-year age range. It requires participants to reproduce the order of a sequence of pictures presented on a computer. To adjust for ability, sequence length varies from 6 to 15 pictures. In the next phase of testing of the instrument (i.e., the norming study), data will be collected that may permit construction of a computerized adapative testing (CAT) version of the test. The data reported in this chapter are the results of validation testing with children ages 3–15 years. Within this age range, the TPSMT is sensitive to age-related changes in learning and episodic memory and also has high test–retest reliability and promising construct validity. The TPSMT thus appears to have strong potential for use in cross-sectional and longitudinal research throughout childhood to early adolescence.

REFERENCES

Adlam, A.-L. R., Vargha-Khadem, F., Mishkin, M., & de Haan, M. (2005). Deferred imitation of action sequences in developmental amnesia. *Journal of Cognitive Neuroscience*, **17**, 240–248.

Arnold, S. E., & Trojanowski, J. Q. (1996). Human fetal hippocampal development: I. Cytoarchitecture, myeloarchitecture, and neuronal morphologic features. *Journal of Comparative Neurology*, **367**, 274–292.

Barbas, H. (2000). Connections underlying the synthesis of cognition, memory, and emotion in primate prefrontal cortices. *Brain Research Bulletin*, **52**, 319–330.

Bauer, P. J. (2005). New developments in the study of infant memory. In D. M. Teti (Ed.), *Blackwell Handbook of research methods in developmental science* (pp. 467–488). Oxford, UK: Blackwell.

Bauer, P. J. (2006). Constructing a past in infancy: A neuro-developmental account. *Trends in Cognitive Sciences*, **10**, 175–181.

Bauer, P. J. (2007). *Remembering the times of our lives: Memory in infancy and beyond*. Mahwah, NJ: Erlbaum.

Bauer, P. J. (2008). Toward a neuro-developmental account of the development of declarative memory. *Developmental Psychobiology*, **50**, 19–31.

Bauer, P. J., Larkina, M., & Deocampo, J. (2011). Early memory development. In U. Goswami (Ed.), *The Wiley-Blackwell handbook of childhood cognitive development* (2nd ed., pp. 153–179). Oxford, UK: Wiley-Blackwell.

Bauer, P. J., & Mandler, J. M. (1989). One thing follows another: Effects of temporal structure on one- to two-year-olds' recall of events. *Developmental Psychology*, **25**, 197–206.

Bauer, P. J., & Shore, C. M. (1987). Making a memorable event: Effects of familiarity and organization on young children's recall of action sequences. *Cognitive Development*, **2**, 327–338.

Bauer, P. J., Wenner, J. A., Dropik, P. L., & Wewerka, S. S. (2000). Parameters of remembering and forgetting in the transition from infancy to early childhood. *Monographs of the Society for Research in Child Development*, **65** (4, Serial No. 263).

Benedict, R. (1997). *Brief visuospatial memory test-revised professional manual.* Odessa, FL: Psychological Assessment Resources.

Benes, F. M. (2001). The development of prefrontal cortex: The maturation of neurotransmitter systems and their interaction. In C. A. Nelson & M. Luciana (Eds.), *Handbook of developmental cognitive neuroscience* (pp. 79–92). Cambridge, MA: MIT Press.

Benes, F. M., Turtle, M., Khan, Y., & Farol, P. (1994). Myelination of a key relay zone in the hippocampal formation occurs in the human brain during childhood, adolescence, and adulthood. *Archives of General Psychiatry,* **51**, 477–484.

Bjorklund, D. F., Dukes, C., & Brown, R. D. (2009). The development of memory strategies. In M. L. Courage & N. Cowan (Eds.), *The developoment of memory in infancy and childhood* (pp. 145–175). New York: Taylor & Francis.

Cabeza, R., Prince, S. E., Daselaar, S. M., Greenberg, D. L., Budde, M., Dolcos, F., et al. (2004). Brain activity during episodic retrieval of autobiographical and laboratory events: An fMRI study using a novel photo paradigm. *Journal of Cognitive Neuroscience,* **16**, 1583–1594.

Churchill, J. D., Stanis, J. J., Press, C., Kushelev, M., & Greenough, W. T. (2003). Is procedural memory relatively spared from age effects? *Neurobiology of Aging,* **24**, 883–892.

Corkin, S. (2002). What's new with the amnesic patient H.M.? *Nature Reviews,* **3**, 153–160.

DeBoer, T., Wewerka, S., Bauer, P. J., Georgieff, M. K., & Nelson, C. A. (2005). Explicit memory performance in infants of diabetic mothers at 1 year of age. *Developmental Medicine and Child Neurology,* **47**, 525–531.

Dunn, L. M., & Dunn, D. M. (2007). *Peabody picture vocabulary test* (4th ed.). San Antonio, TX: Pearson.

Eichenbaum, H., & Cohen, N. J. (2001). *From conditioning to conscious recollection: Memory systems of the brain.* New York: Oxford University Press.

Fuster, J. M. (2002). Frontal lobe and cognitive development. *Journal of Neurocytology,* **31**, 373–385.

Gadian, D. G., Aicardi, J., Watkins, K. E., Porter, D. A., Mishkin, M., & Vargha-Khadem, F. (2000). Developmental amnesia associated with hear hypoxic-ischaemic injury. *Brain,* **123**, 499–507.

Gogtay, N., Giedd, J. N., Lusk, L., Hayashi, K. M., Greenstein, D., Vaituzis, A. C., et al. (2004). Dynamic mapping of human cortical development during childhood through early adulthood. *Proceedings of the National Academy of Science United States of America,* **101**, 8174–8179.

Huttenlocher, P. R. (1979). Synaptic density in human frontal cortex: Developmental changes and effects of aging. *Brain Research,* **163**, 195–205.

Huttenlocher, P. R., & Dabholkar, A. S. (1997). Regional differences in synaptogenesis in human cerebral cortex. *Journal of Comparative Neurology,* **387**, 167–178.

Korkman, M., Kork, U., & Kemp, S. (2007). *NEPSY-II* (2nd ed.). San Antonio, TX: Harcourt Assessment.

Maguire, E. A. (2001). Neuroimaging studies of autobiographical event memory. *Philosophical Transactions of the Royal Society of London,* **356**, 1441–1451.

McGaugh, J. L. (2000). Memory—A century of consolidation. *Science,* **287**, 248–251.

Menon, V., Boyett-Anderson, J. M., & Reiss, A. L. (2005). Maturation of medial temporal lobe response and connectivity during memory encoding. *Cognitive Brain Research,* **25**, 379–385.

Ofen, N., Kao, Y.-C., Sokol-Hessner, P., Kim, H., Whitfield-Gabrieli, S., & Gabrieli, J. D. E. (2007). Development of the declarative memory system in the human brain. *Nature Neuroscience*, **10**, 1198–1205.

Olesen, P. J., Nagy, Z., Westerberg, H., & Klingberg, T. (2003). Combined analysis of DTI and fMRI data reveals a joint maturation of white and grey matter in a fronto-parietal network. *Cognitive Brain Research*, **18**, 48–57.

Petrides, M. (1995). Impairments on nonspatial self-ordered and externally ordered working memory tasks after lesions of the mid-dorsal part of the lateral frontal cortex in monkeys. *The Journal of Neuroscience*, **15**, 359–375.

Pfluger, T., Weil, S., Wies, S., Vollmar, C., Heiss, D., Egger, J., et al. (1999). Normative volumetric data of the developing hippocampus in children based on magnetic resonance imaging. *Epilepsia*, **40**, 414–423.

Reber, P. J., Martinez, L. A., & Weintraub, S. (2003). Artificial grammar learning in Alzheimer's disease. *Cognitive Affective Behavioral Neuroscience*, **3**, 145–153.

Riggins, T., Miller, N. C., Bauer, P. J., Georgieff, M. K., Nelson, C. A. (2009). Consequences of low neonatal iron status due to maternal diabetes mellitus on explicit memory performance in childhood. *Developmental Neuropsychology*, **34**, 762–779.

Schneider, J. F. L., Il'yasov, K. A., Hennig, J., & Martin, E. (2004). Fast quantitative difusion-tensor imaging of cerebral white matter from the neonatal period to adolescence. *Neuroradiology*, **46**, 258–266.

Shimamura, A. P., Janowsky, J. S., & Squire, L. R. (1990). Memory for the temporal order of events in patients with frontal lobe lesions and amnesic patients. *Neuropsychologia*, **28**, 803–813.

Sowell, E. R., Delis, D., Stiles, J., & Jernigan, T. L. (2001). Improved memory functioning and frontal lobe maturation between childhood and adolescence: A structural MRI study. *Journal of International Neuropsychological Society*, **7**, 312–322.

Squire, L. R. (2004). Memory systems of the brain: A brief history and current perspective. *Neurobiology of Learning and Memory*, **82**, 171–177.

Squire, L. R., Knowlton, B., & Musen, G. (1993). The structure and organization of memory. *Annual Review of Psychology*, **44**, 453–495.

Strauss, E., Sherman, E. M. S., & Spreen, O. (2006). *A compendium of neuropsychological tests: Administration, norms, and commentary*. New York: Oxford University Press.

Tulving, E. (2000). Concepts of memory. In E. Tulving & F. I. M. Craik (Eds.), *The Oxford handbook of memory* (pp. 33–42). New York: Oxford University Press.

Utsunomiya, H., Takano, K., Okazaki, M., & Mistudome, A. (1999). Development of the temporal lobe in infants and children: Analysis by MR-based volumetry. *American Journal of Neuroradiology*, **20**, 717–723.

Weintraub, S., Dikmen, S. S., Heaton, R. K., Tulsky, D. S., Zelazo, P. D., Bauer, P. J., et al. (2013). NIH Toolbox for the assessment of behavioral and neurological function: Cognition domain instruments. *Neurology*, **80**, S54–S64.

Zola, S. M., & Squire, L. R. (2000). The medial temporal lobe and the hippocampus. In E. Tulving & F. I. M. Craik (Eds.), *The Oxford handbook of memory* (pp. 485–500). New York: Oxford University Press.

IV. NIH TOOLBOX COGNITION BATTERY (CB): MEASURING LANGUAGE (VOCABULARY COMPREHENSION AND READING DECODING)

Richard C. Gershon, Jerry Slotkin, Jennifer J. Manly, David L. Blitz, Jennifer L. Beaumont, Deborah Schnipke, Kathleen Wallner-Allen, Roberta Michnick Golinkoff, Jean Berko Gleason, Kathy Hirsh-Pasek, Marilyn Jager Adams, and Sandra Weintraub

ABSTRACT Mastery of language skills is an important predictor of daily functioning and health. Vocabulary comprehension and reading decoding are relatively quick and easy to measure and correlate highly with overall cognitive functioning, as well as with success in school and work. New measures of vocabulary comprehension and reading decoding (in both English and Spanish) were developed for the NIH Toolbox Cognition Battery (CB). In the Toolbox Picture Vocabulary Test (TPVT), participants hear a spoken word while viewing four pictures, and then must choose the picture that best represents the word. This approach tests receptive vocabulary knowledge without the need to read or write, removing the literacy load for children who are developing literacy and for adults who struggle with reading and writing. In the Toolbox Oral Reading Recognition Test (TORRT), participants see a letter or word onscreen and must pronounce or identify it. The examiner determines whether it was pronounced correctly by comparing the response to the pronunciation guide on a separate computer screen. In this chapter, we discuss the importance of language during childhood and the relation of language and brain function. We also review the development of the TPVT and TORRT, including information about the item calibration process and results from a validation study. Finally, the strengths and weaknesses of the measures are discussed.

In this chapter, we discuss language as represented by measures of vocabulary comprehension and reading decoding (in both English and Spanish) in the Cognition Battery (CB) of the NIH Toolbox for the Assessment of Neurological and Behavioral Function (Gershon et al., 2010).

Corresponding author: Sandra Weintraub, Cognitive Neurology and Alzheimer's Disease Center, Northwestern Feinberg School of Medicine, 303 E Chicago, IL 60611, email: sweintraub@northwestern.edu

Subdomain Definition

Language is a shared symbol system that facilitates communication, categorization, and thought (Pinker, 2000). The simplest definition of language is that it is a means of communication consisting of all the words used by a community and the rules for varying and combining them. Language users can express the full range of their experience by joining words into clauses, sentences, and connected discourse (Gleason & Ratner, 2009). Language can be spoken or written, or it can be transmitted gesturally, as in sign language. Though language does not require audition and speech (as in sign language), important language abilities include auditory comprehension, speaking, naming, reading, and writing. Language is hierarchically organized, and composed of a number of subsystems. These include phonology, morphology, syntax, the lexicon and semantics, pragmatics, and discourse—components that have been linked to constituents within a large-scale neuroanatomical network primarily in the left cerebral hemisphere (Price, 2000).

Communication via spoken and written language promotes the transmission of culture, societal values, and history. In an ever more literate world, language skills are important predictors of daily functioning and health (Burton, Strauss, Hultsch, & Hunter, 2006). Language is commonly assessed through receptive vocabulary (comprehension), expressive vocabulary and production, object naming, speech fluency, reading, and writing.

For purposes of the NIH Toolbox CB, it was desirable to establish quick measures, available for researchers' use at low or no cost, that would correlate highly with overall cognitive functioning and with success in school and work (Kastner, May, & Hildman, 2001; Schmidt & Hunter, 2004). Vocabulary comprehension was chosen as the primary language measure after much deliberation and with the full recognition of the equivalent importance of grammatical proficiency for development and growth (Gleason & Ratner, 2009; Hirsh-Pasek & Golinkoff, 1996). Vocabulary knowledge is of particular interest because it has a high association with general measures of "intelligence," or the "g" factor (Cattell, 1987) and with success in school and work (Kastner et al., 2001; Schmidt & Hunter, 2004).

The TORRT, the second language measure, is a proxy for a broad range of cognitive, educational, and socioeconomic factors. The ability to pronounce low-frequency words with irregular orthography has also been used as an estimate of overall intelligence (Grober & Sliwinski, 1991). The TORRT measures the accuracy of pronouncing single printed words and of naming or recognizing single letters. In healthy individuals, single-word reading tasks reflect (1) level of exposure to written text/material; (2) whether one's environment provided a context in which to develop basic and complex reading skills; (3) specific cognitive skills needed to develop decoding, such as phonological processing and working memory; and (4) general cognitive ability, since more "able" individuals are expected to be exposed to a greater volume and higher complexity of written stimuli.

Importance During Childhood

Language consists of a complex system of rules that is acquired relatively effortlessly by infants. Children across a wide range of different environments and cultures learn to understand and use language in a remarkably short period of time. Language has a biological basis. It depends both on skills specific to language (e.g., the perception of phonemes) and general cognitive skills (e.g., categorization and memory) (Kuhl & Rivera-Gaxiola, 2008). Comprehension of single words is a fundamental language skill that infants begin to acquire well before children speak (Kuhl, 2004). Infants typically have a repertoire of about 50 words they can understand before age 1 year (Fenson et al., 1994) and typically begin to produce single word utterances around their first birthdays. Typically, they begin to combine words to form brief sentences by the age of 2 years. Initially syntax is highly simplified, but over time develops to include more complex constructions. For example, reversible passive sentences like "Bart was seen by Marge" are not correctly comprehended at a 90% level until age 9 (Hirsch & Wexler, 2007). Acquisition of basic letter and word recognition skills typically begins in preschool and is typically well anchored by second grade. Over the ensuing school years, through instruction and practice in reading and writing, children's ability to read and spell words continues to grow and to become richly interconnected with their development of vocabulary and grammatical knowledge.

Writing is the last major language skill to emerge in early childhood. In young children, measures of language function need to capture proficiency in comprehension, naming, and generating and interpreting simple sentences. As the fundamental skills become more established in late childhood and early adolescence, vocabulary increases and language becomes the primary medium for establishing and accessing "semantic memory"—our storehouse of information and facts. In young adulthood and into old age, vocabulary and semantic memory are referred to as "crystallized capacities" that are relatively resistant to the effects of aging and neurological disease (see Heaton et al., Chapter 8, this volume; National Research Council Committee on the Prevention of Reading Difficulties in Young Children, Snow, Burns, Griffin, & National Research Council Commission on Behavioral Social Sciences Education, 2002; Sternberg, 2004). Reading encompasses phonological, orthographic, and semantic processing, and several models have been proposed to account for reading ability (National Early Literacy Panel & National Center for Family Literacy, 2008; National Research Council Committee on the Prevention of Reading Difficulties in Young Children et al., 2002).

To build rapid and functional word recognition skills, beginning readers must first develop basic language and decoding skills (National Reading Panel & National Institute of Child Health and Human Development, 2000). Reading also demands a modicum of world experience and vocabulary knowledge so that children can begin to use reading to learn, which typically takes place at the third grade level (Dickinson, Golinkoff, & Hirsh-Pasek, 2010).

The process of sounding out words results in neural associations between letters or graphemes and the phonemes they represent. As readers repeatedly encounter common sequences of letters, these associations become extended and differentiated, linking larger spelling patterns with larger phonological units and resulting in what is known as *decoding automaticity*—the ability to pronounce even new and less familiar words quickly, easily, and accurately provided that they are regularly spelled. Irregular words (e.g., "one," "two," "colonel," and "island"), whose spelling-sound correspondences do not conform to the norms of the language, become set off and learned as wholes. Repeated experience reading and decoding sequences of letters that correspond to the same "phoneme blend" allow the reader to build a knowledge base that can be applied to correctly pronounce words. However, irregular words, whose pronunciations do not conform to the rules, require different lexical routes for correct pronunciation. The ability to read regularly versus irregularly spelled words is differentially affected among people with acquired dyslexia due to brain trauma (Rapcsak, Henry, Teague, Carnahan, & Beeson, 2007; Ziegler et al., 2008).

Developmental disorders of language and communication (e.g., autism, dyslexia) and limited opportunities to acquire literacy in childhood have a significant impact on academic achievement and life adaptation in developed countries. Scores on language measures can predict occupational attainment and performance (Schmidt & Hunter, 2004). Many acquired conditions can affect language in adulthood, including stroke and Alzheimer's disease (Kastner et al., 2001).

There is evidence that reading disability may be under-identified in children if measures of reading fluency, such as naming speed, are not included (Meisinger, Bloom, & Hynd, 2010). Single-word reading recognition tasks are strong predictors of health and cognition outcomes across the lifespan. Poor health literacy (literacy skills related to health information, such as reading prescription bottles, appointment slips, or medical education brochures) is one critical factor in health outcome, especially in older adults (Wolf, Gazmararian, & Baker, 2005). Performance on single-word reading recognition tasks is also useful as a general estimate of reading level and quality of education (Manly, Byrd, Touradji, & Stern, 2004; Manly et al., 1999).

Relation of Subdomain With Brain Function

From a clinical perspective, language capabilities are sometimes divided into two broad categories: receptive language and expressive language. Receptive language involves the comprehension of language. Expressive language involves the production of language and includes skills such as naming, speaking, and repeating. Although this is a convenient way to divide language functions for the clinician, on a cognitive systems level, language is not represented in that manner. Instead, the psycholinguistically supported subcomponents of language are its phonology (or basic sound system), morphology (structure of words and their modifiers), lexicon (the dictionary of all words in any given language), syntax (the rules of grammar that link words together), and semantics (meaning) (Gleason, 1997). Speakers who have communicative competence must also be aware of discourse rules that govern the way that utterances may be combined, as well as pragmatic rules for appropriate language in social settings. It is these components of language that are represented in the brain in the context of a language system, rather than merely the dichotomy of input and output capabilities.

Early evidence supporting that the left cerebral hemisphere of the brain is the major contributor to language functions came from the study of patients who had suffered strokes in various regions of the left perisylvian area. Classical models of aphasiology were based on this type of evidence. Different aphasia subtypes correspond to the loss of one or more components of language. Thus, patients with strokes can be agrammatic, having difficulty comprehending and producing small grammatical features of language while others can produce normal grammar but have difficulty accessing nouns and verbs. In more recent years, studies of nonbrain-injured individuals using functional neuroimaging have affirmed the relative modularity of language components (Caplan & Hildebrandt, 1988; Friederici, Rüschemeyer, Hahne, & Fiebach, 2003; Price, 1998).

To assess the language subdomain, we developed the TPVT and the TORRT. To develop these new measures and assess their psychometric properties, we adhered to stringent development processes and utilized state-of-the-art psychometric approaches, in an effort to assess whether researchers will obtain stable and valid scores when using these measures. A detailed description of these processes is provided below.

METHOD

Participants

Two samples of participants were used in the preliminary item calibration for the TPVT. The goal of the calibration sample was to calculate item response theory parameters for the item bank. Matching participant vocabulary ability with item difficulty was of primary importance in calibration accrual. The first sample contained 4,703 participants ranging in age from 3 to 69 ($n = 3{,}190$ children ages 3–17, Mean = 9.41, Female = 48.1%; $n = 1{,}513$ adults ages 18–69, Mean = 25.76, Female = 61.1%), with education for adults spread relatively evenly from completion of 10th grade through graduate/doctorate level. Participants were recruited via an online panel company (a company that specializes in procuring subjects for online surveys and test administrations), and participants were paid to take the test online. Parents of children under age 7 years were given specific instructions about how to administer the test to their children, what their children would be asked to do, and how to help children maintain attention and complete the tests without providing material assistance. Participants were administered one of 21 test forms that were believed to closely match their likely ability level (based on age for those 17 years and under and based on level of education for participants 18 years and above).

Unlike the TPVT, online calibration testing for the TORRT was not an option, given the requirement for one-on-one administration (after the participant reads the item on the screen the test administrator scores the item right or wrong). Instead, 146 participants for the initial item calibrations were recruited from the general population from four geographic locations to test at five sites associated with some of our academic collaborators: West Orange, NJ; Minneapolis, MN; Atlanta, GA; Evanston, IL; and Chicago, IL. The data from these participants were used in the initial item calibrations. Data from the validation study (see Weintraub et al., Chapter 1, and Table 3, this volume, for sample composition) were combined with those from the data collection described above. This merged sample was then used to recalibrate items prior to use in the norming study.

The sample from which the validation results discussed in this chapter were derived is described in Weintraub et al. (Chapter 1, this volume; Table 2).

Measures

Toolbox Picture Vocabulary Test (TPVT)

For the TPVT, single words are presented via an audio file, paired simultaneously with four images of objects, actions, and/or depictions of concepts (e.g., ball, running, friendship; see Figure 6). The participant is asked to select the picture whose meaning most closely corresponds with the spoken word. Participants are permitted as much time as necessary to complete their responses. Because the test does not require reading or writing, the test design removes the literacy load for children and for those who struggle with literacy skills. Further, the test does not require a spoken response, making it particularly suitable for children.

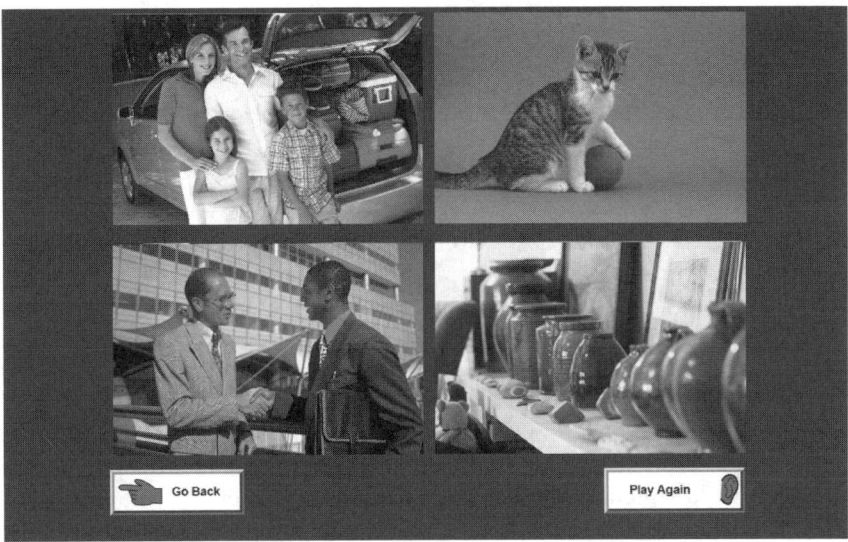

FIGURE 6.—Sample item from the Toolbox Picture Vocabulary Test ("Kin").
Note. Photo Credits (clockwise from upper left): Flying Colours Ltd/Photodisc/Getty Images; David De Lossy/Photodisc/Getty Images; Stockbyte/Getty Images; Andy Sotiriou/Photodisc/Getty Images.

To select words, initial candidate words were based on difficulty, from previously field-tested and calibrated items made available by the Johnson-O'Connor Research Foundation (Gershon, 1988). Additional items were drawn from the *Living Word Vocabulary* (Dale & O'Rourke, 1976) and *Children's Writer's Word Book* (Mogilner, 1992) based on the need for age, difficulty level, and frequency. Candidate words were then reviewed against the University of Western Australia MRC Psycholinguistic Database (UWASP, 2011) to evaluate how well they could potentially be translated into a photograph. Words with low imageability were dropped from the list of candidates. The list of potential words was then reviewed by experts (a diverse group of pediatric and geriatric professionals with "language expertise") and pruned accordingly based upon their feedback.

To create distractors for each item (word), four answer options were written, and these functioned as requirements for photographs that were eventually selected. The distractors all needed to be plausible but incorrect and had to have high imageability as described above, so that photos could eventually be selected as the corresponding answer choices. A senior internal content team then reviewed all items; modifications were made resulting in the deletion of a small number of additional items. Items were then re-reviewed by the language experts for content and sensitivity, with specific instruction that these descriptions would be the basis for photo selection and then subsequent reviews. Items and distractors were further modified or dropped based on expert feedback, and prepared for the photo selection process.

Color photographs for the four options for each item of the TPVT (one correct answer and three distractors) were selected from the Getty Images library of millions of high-quality, photographic images. Initially, Getty staff provided 4–10 suggested images for each of the item options. The senior content team at Northwestern University, together with the language experts, were then trained in photo selection, and an extensive review process was implemented to ensure appropriate photos were selected. The selection process included a review by a multicultural group of experts empaneled to view all items for fairness and sensitivity. Items were edited or dropped based on the group's feedback. In many cases, the reviewers went back to the database and searched for additional photographs that would better meet the needs for any given item. Photos selected were then edited professionally where needed, primarily to make photos more consistent in background and orientation within a given item and to remove extraneous information in selected photos.

Item Calibration

In the preliminary item calibration for TPVT, each participant was administered 40–60 items from the pool of 625 items (children under age 8 years were generally administered the shorter, 40-item forms). Forms utilized common items (each form shared 50% of the items with its adjacent form) to allow for successful equating across forms. Each item received approximately 200 unique administrations to participants. Items were scored right/wrong and were calibrated using the one-parameter/Rasch Item Response Theory model (Rasch, 1960) as analyzed using Winsteps (Linacre, 2005).

Based on the initial analysis, items were reordered by difficulty and misfitting items were removed, leaving 602 items from which to construct an initial item bank to enable initial computer adaptive testing (CAT) for use in the validation study. A fixed-length 25-item CAT was constructed. A fixed-length strategy was used over a typical variable length CAT with a standard-error cutoff. This strategy "forced" participants to take a total of 25 items (versus fewer, which might be expected with the variable length test) in order to oversample items, allowing for the accumulation of additional data to refine the item calibrations. The difficulty of each successive item presented is based on the current estimate of the participant's ability level, as estimated by their responses to the previously administered items on the test. Items were administered to match each participant's ability with item difficulty, with the consequence that each participant was correct on approximately 50% of the items. (Final target percentage correct will be adjusted based on norming to enable younger participants to have a higher "success" experience, to improve motivation.) The average administration time was about 5 min.

Toolbox Oral Reading Recognition Test

For the TORRT, a word or letter is presented on the computer screen, and the participant is asked to read it aloud. Participants are permitted as much time as necessary to complete their responses. Responses are recorded as correct or incorrect by the examiner, who views accepted pronunciations on a separate computer screen. A sample TORRT item is shown in Figure 7, with the participant screen shown in Panel (a) and the examiner screen shown in Panel (b) (Toolbox examiners must be trained on correct word pronunciation prior to administering this measure). For "prereaders" and those with low literacy levels, letters and other multiple-choice "prereading" items are presented, making the test as accessible as possible for young children. "Ceiling" rules were also implemented to minimize frustration, especially for early and prereaders.

Initial candidate words were drawn from the University of Western Australia MRC Psycholinguistic Database (UWASP, 2011). A variety of search criteria were applied, including frequency in the language, complexity of letter-sound relations, orthographical typicality, age of acquisition rating, number of syllables, and number of phonemes. Individual letters of the alphabet were later added to this list to enable assessment of emerging reading ability.

The Kucera and Francis rating (Kucera & Francis, 1967), which is closely correlated with Brown Verbal Frequency (Brown, 1984), was the frequency statistic that was present most often in the database. Many words had no Kucera and Francis frequency information, however, which indicates that they were not present in that corpus (low frequency). The letters and words were selected using the following guidelines: (1) letters could be roughly matched in relative frequency with another letter in the alphabet; (2) words had between 2 and 14 letters; (3) within words with 2–4 letters, emphasis was placed on including frequent words (for words with 5 or more letters, a few common words were included but this was not emphasized); (4) among words with 5 or more letters, a sample of words with low Kucera and Francis frequency was selected; (5) among words with 4 or more letters, a sample of words with an irregular orthography to phonology match, regardless of frequency, was selected; (6) words that appeared to be technical terms (e.g., medical or zoological terms) were eschewed; (7) words with many different acceptable pronunciations were avoided for ease of scoring.

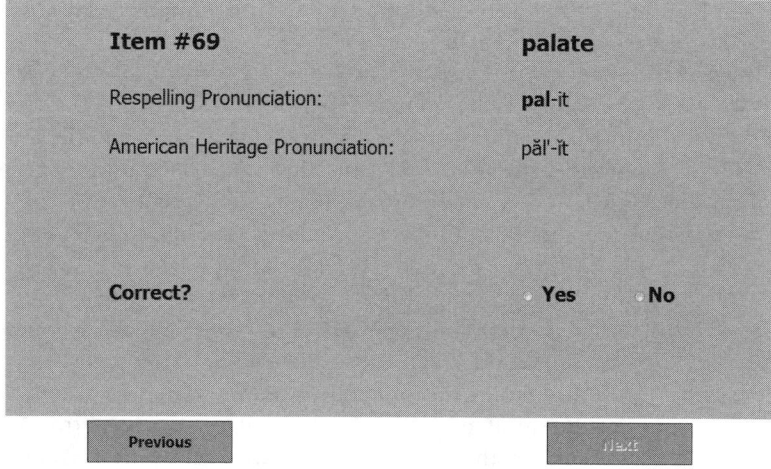

FIGURE 7.—Sample item from the Toolbox Oral Reading Recognition Test. The participant's screen is shown in Panel a, and the examiner's screen is shown in Panel b.

National experts in reading as well as a diverse group with expertise in language and pediatrics or geriatrics reviewed the initial word list. Words were eliminated or added based on experts' feedback, resulting in an initial item pool of 268 words and 21 letters and prereading items. The prereading items were developed in a multiple-choice format in which the respondent is asked, for example, to identify the letter when shown three nonletter symbols and a letter, or to identify a specific letter (e.g., "B") when three other letters (or nonletter symbols) are shown.

A subset of items with an expected broad range of difficulty was pilot tested to determine what format to use for the test. Two 50-item forms designed to be parallel in length and frequency of words were created; one form was administered one item per screen, and the other had 5–6 items per screen. Each form took 5 min or less for participants. Given that both forms took a similar length of time, the format with one item per screen (easier for the examiner to score and less cluttered for the participant), was selected for the test.

Item Calibration

For the item calibration, a 9-item screener was used to determine which test form the respondent would receive. Four test forms were created from 280 items, with the following numbers of items per form: Form 1 (70 items); Form 2 (101 items); Form 3 (120 items); and Form 4 (125 items). Based on rough preliminary information, it was expected that Form 1 would be easier than Form 2, which was expected to be easier than Form 3, etc. Each form had approximately one-third common items to allow for successful calibration.

The 9-item screener was administered to participants aged 8 years and older; participants aged 3–7 years did not receive the screener and immediately proceeded to Form 1. Based on performance on the routing form, older children (and adults) received one of the four forms. Prior to administration, brief instructions were read to the participant. For the screener and all forms, items were presented in dual-screen mode, whereby the participant was presented the word on one screen and the examiner was presented with a scoring template and phonetic key on the other screen. Participants attempted items until they either finished the prescribed number of items for their form or they mispronounced 10 words in a row (the discontinue rule used for calibration).

For the validation study, each participant was again administered one of four forms as described above, so that a fuller calibration of the 289 items could be achieved. Results were combined with the previous data set for calibration, and were analyzed separately for the purposes of assessing convergent and discriminant validity. The average administration time was 6 min.

Validation Measures

Peabody Picture Test-4th Edition (PPVT-IV) (Dunn & Dunn, 2007)

The PPVT-IV is a test of receptive vocabulary that is individually administered and provides an estimate of verbal ability or scholastic aptitude. The test is given verbally and takes 10–15 min to administer. For its administration, the examiner presents a series of pictures (four to a page) to the test taker. Stating a word describing one of the pictures, the examiner asks the participant to point to or say the number of the picture they feel best corresponds to the word. The total score can be converted to a percentile rank, mental age, or a standard deviation IQ score. The test is available in two parallel forms of 228 items each. Internal consistency coefficients across ages are .94 for each alternate form; test–retest reliability is .93. The PPVT-IV was used as a measure of convergent validity for the TPVT.

Wide Range Achievement Test Version 4-Reading Subtest (WRAT-IV) (Wilkinson & Robertson, 2006)

The WRAT-IV is an individually administered test in which test takers are asked to name letters and read aloud words out of context. The words are listed in order of decreasing familiarity and increasing phonological complexity. Median internal consistency coefficients across ages for each of the alternate forms used individually range from .87 to .96. Alternate-form immediate retest reliability coefficients range from .78 to .89 for an age-based sample. Validity evidence for the WRAT-IV is derived from the content and structure of the test battery, studies with special groups, and correlations with other widely used achievement and cognitive ability measures. Standard scores, percentiles, stanines, normal curve equivalents, and Rasch scaled scores are provided for the WRAT-IV. Note that although the WRAT-IV is not ordinarily administered below age 5, we did so for comparison purposes and correlated the raw scores for each measure. The WRAT-IV was included primarily to serve as a measure of convergent validity for the TORRT.

Brief Visuospatial Memory Test-Revised (BVMT-R Total Recall) (Benedict, 1997)

The BVMT-R is designed to measure visuospatial memory. Participants view six geometric figures on a page and are asked to draw as many of the figures as possible from memory in their correct location, after the figures are removed from view. Reliability coefficients range from .96 to .97 for the three Learning trials, .97 for Total Recall, and .97 for Delayed Recall. Test–retest reliability coefficients range from .60 for Trial 1 to .84 for Trial 3. The BVMT-R correlates most strongly with other tests of visual memory and less strongly with tests of verbal memory. The BVMT-R was included to serve as an assessment of discriminant validity for both CB Language tests and was administered only to ages 8 and up.

Rey Auditory Verbal Learning Test (RAVLT) (Rey, 1958)

The RAVLT starts with a list of 15 words, read aloud by the examiner at the rate of one word per second. The participant's task is to repeat as many words as possible, in any order. This procedure was carried out a total of three times in comparison with the usual five trials conducted in the standard administration. The RAVLT was also included as a measure of discriminant validity for the TPVT and was administered to ages 8 years and up.

Analyses

Normalized scaled scores were used for all analyses. These scores were created by first ranking the test scores, next applying a normative transformation to the ranks to create a standard normal distribution, and finally rescaling the distribution to have a mean of 10 and a standard deviation of 3. Pearson correlation coefficients between age and test performance were calculated to assess the ability of the NIH Toolbox language tests to detect cognitive developmental growth during childhood. Intraclass correlation coefficients (*ICC*) with 95% confidence intervals were calculated to evaluate test–retest reliability. Convergent validity was assessed with correlations between each CB measure and an established measure of the same construct (PPVT-IV for Vocabulary and WRAT-IV for Reading). Evidence of discriminant validity consisted of lower correlations with selected measures of a *different* cognitive construct (BVMT-R and RAVLT) for both TPVT and TORRT.

RESULTS (TPVT)

Eight children did not successfully complete the TPVT for reasons such as lack of attention or alertness or general noncompliance.

Age Effects

Age was significantly correlated with the TPVT score ($n = 200$; $r = .81$; $p < .001$), as well as the PPVT-IV ($n = 201$; $r = .88$; $p < .001$). A quadratic model provided the best fit of the data, with $R^2 = .67$. Pairwise comparisons between age groups are reported in Appendix. In the subset of participants age 3–6 years, the correlation between TPVT and age was .42 ($n = 112$, $p < .001$). In participants age 8 to 15 years, the correlation was .57 ($n = 88$, $p < .001$). Figure 8 shows TPVT scores as a function of age. It should be noted that the TPVT and PPVT-IV scores closely mimic each other at every age level.

Test–Retest Reliability

The test–retest reliability of the TPVT was $ICC = .81$ ($n = 66$; 95% confidence interval: .71, .88). Reliability of the PPVT-IV in our sample was $ICC = .96$ ($n = 65$; 95% confidence interval: .94, .98).

Effect of Repeated Testing

Practice effects were computed as the difference between test and retest normalized scaled scores, with significance of the effect being tested with *t*

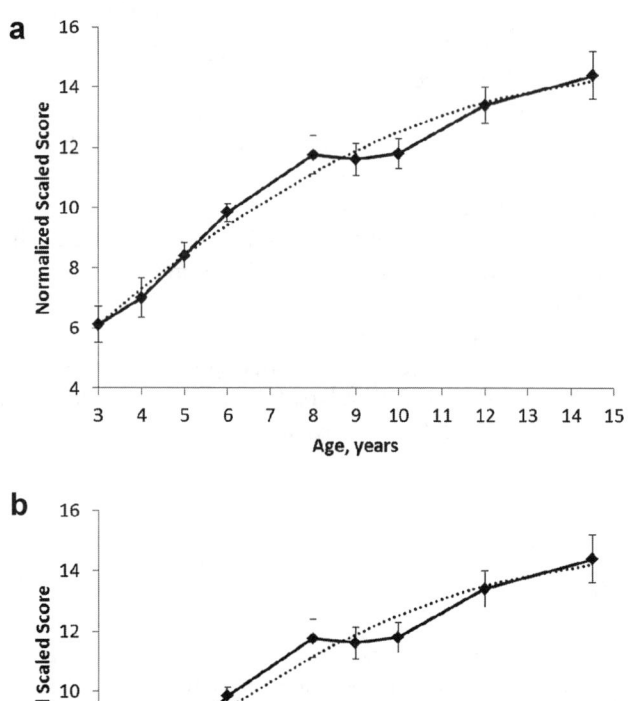

FIGURE 8.—Normalized scaled scores on the Toolbox Picture Vocabulary Test (A) and the Toolbox Oral Reading Recognition Test (B) across age groups. Error bars are ±2 standard errors. Best-fitting polynomial curves are also shown (see text).

tests for dependent means. For the total child group (ages 3–15 years, $n = 66$), the TPVT showed no practice effect over an average 2-week test–retest interval: *mean practice effect* = .1, SD = 1.79, $t(65)$ = .43, p = .67.

Criterion Validity

Convergent and Discriminant Validity

Table 8 shows the correlations with the validation measures for ages 3–15 years. The TPVT scores correlated well with the PPVT-IV, which taps the same construct, thus providing evidence of excellent convergent validity. The TPVT

TABLE 8

PEARSON CORRELATIONS BETWEEN TOOLBOX VOCABULARY COMPREHENSION SCORES AND VALIDATION MEASURES

	N	r	p-Value
PPVT-IV	198	.90	<.001
BVMT-R Total Recall	87	.46	<.001
RAVLT	85	.42	<.001
Average of BVMT-R Total Recall and RAVLT	87	.53	<.001

Note. WRAT-IV, Wide Range Achievement Test-4th Edition; PPVT-IV, Peabody Picture Vocabulary Test-4th Edition; BVMT-R, Brief Visuospatial Memory Test-Revised; RAVLT, Rey Auditory Verbal Learning Test. © 2006–2012 National Institutes of Health and Northwestern University.

score correlated weakly with measures that tap different constructs (the BVMT-R Total Recall, RAVLT, and the average of BVMT-R Total Recall and RAVLT), providing evidence of discriminant validity. The discriminant correlations were significantly lower than the convergent correlations ($p < .003$).

RESULTS (TORRT)

Four children did not successfully complete the TORRT for reasons such as lack of attention or alertness or general noncompliance.

Age Effects

Age was significantly correlated with the TORRT score ($n = 204$; $r = .86$; $p < .001$), as well as the WRAT-IV ($n = 203$; $r = .88$; $p < .001$). A quadratic model provided the best fit of the data, with $R^2 = .78$. Pairwise comparisons between age groups are reported in Appendix A. In the subset of participants age 3–6 the correlation between TORRT and age was .73 ($n = 117, p < .001$). In participants age 8–15 the correlation was .64 ($n = 87, p < .001$). Figure 8 shows TORRT scores as a function of age. It should be noted that TORRT scores and WRAT scores almost mirror each other at every age.

Test–Retest Reliability

The test–retest reliability for the TORRT was $ICC = .97$ ($n = 65$; 95% confidence interval: .95, .98). Reliability for the WRAT-IV was $ICC = .96$ ($n = 65$; 95% confidence interval: .94, .98).

Effect of Repeated Testing

Practice effects were computed as the difference between test and retest normalized scaled scores, with significance of the effect being tested with t

tests for dependent means. For the total child group (ages 3–15 years, $n = 66$), the TORRT showed no practice effect over an average 2-week test–retest interval: *mean practice effect* $= -.05$, $SD = .80$, $t(64) = -.51$, $p = .61$.

Criterion Validity

Convergent and Discriminant Validity

Table 9 shows the correlations with the validation measures for ages 3–15 years. The TORRT scores correlated well with WRAT-IV, which taps the same construct, providing evidence of excellent convergent validity, and weakly with the measure that taps a different construct (the BVMT-R Total Recall, which as previously noted was only administered to ages 8 and up), providing evidence of discriminant validity. The discriminant correlations were significantly lower than the convergent correlations ($p < .001$). The correlation between the TORRT scores and PPVT-IV scores was moderate, confirming the known relation between reading and vocabulary, but also providing evidence of the independence of the two constructs.

DISCUSSION

Development of the NIH Toolbox Picture Vocabulary Test and the NIH Toolbox Oral Reading Recognition Test represents an unprecedented effort to create high-quality language assessments using cutting edge psychometric theory and computer-based test administration. We have demonstrated that precise assessments of each of these constructs can be obtained in 5 min with a level of accuracy not seen in any other short assessment of this kind. Ceiling and floor effects, common to most measures covering a wide range of ability,

TABLE 9

PEARSON CORRELATIONS BETWEEN TOOLBOX ORAL READING RECOGNITION SCORES AND VALIDATION MEASURES

	N	r	p-Value
WRAT-IV	202	.96	<.0001
PPVT-IV	200	.87	<.0001
BVMT-R Total Recall	86	.41	<.0001
RAVLT	84	.45	<.0001
Average of BVMT-R Total Recall and RAVLT	86	.53	<.0001

Note. WRAT-IV, Wide Range Achievement Test-4th Edition; PPVT-IV, Peabody Picture Vocabulary Test-4th Edition; BVMT-R, Brief Visuospatial Memory Test-Revised; RAVLT, Rey Auditory Verbal Learning Test. © 2006–2012 National Institutes of Health and Northwestern University.

have been removed through the inclusion of a large corpus of items, spanning the complete continuum of difficulty, from preemerging language through PhD-level materials. An advantage of all computer adaptive measures is that the reliability can be estimated for each individual participant and not just as an "average" across the total sample (the typical measure of reliability cited for fixed-length instruments). This enables the researcher to individually assess the accuracy of the measure obtained.

Each measure has been reduced to as pure a form as possible. The TPVT has no reading component and is prompted by listening to a professionally recorded voice. The TORRT presents simple letter or word prompts on a clear field background with no distractions. TPVT has several advantages over the PPVT, including the increased sensitivity that results from having more words at every level, particularly at higher ability levels.

The photographic prompts for the vocabulary items are both contemporary and appealing. These professional images have been licensed for research use in perpetuity. Licensing for higher resolutions was also acquired, insuring continued use with evolving technology. As common monitor resolutions continue to improve (e.g., yesterday's VGA standard versus today's high definition), the NIH Toolbox items can be re-released in higher resolution formats.

The test–retest correlation as well as convergent and discriminant validity results obtained for both CB language measures were strong. The relation of each measure to participant age was as expected. Test–retest reliability for the PPVT-IV was noted to be stronger than that obtained with the TPVT, implying that the accuracy of the CB scores obtained were marginally weaker. This may be attributable to the fact that the CB measures were designed to be administered in 5 min, as compared to the PPVT-IV, which has administration times reported to fall in the 10–15 min range. Generally, a longer, well-developed test will always outperform a shorter one. Given the goal to create a "brief" measure of language proficiency for use in the NIH Toolbox, the newly created vocabulary comprehension measure performs admirably. For researchers who require increased reliability (as might be the case when examining individual ability at a clinical level), the CAT algorithm can be adjusted to administer a longer test. Clinical level accuracy can similarly be obtained for the TORRT through adjustment of the reading CAT algorithm. Additionally, TPVT responding during validation was through the use of a touch screen—a modality judged to be poor for the youngest children. During the NIH Toolbox norming phase, young children will be directed to point to the correct answer or use a mouse.

The vocabulary measure within CB is largely patterned after vocabulary measures that have been used in the past to infer more general linguistic attainment. These tests, such as the PPVT-IV or the Picture Vocabulary measure on the Woodcock–Johnson-III, are weighted toward nouns and object words, and test vocabulary knowledge (vs. grammatical competence). As a practical matter, we were constrained to use vocabulary as the primary index of language. Time and delivery method precluded development of an assessment that measured multiple language skills. We also wrestled with these constraints, knowing that full language competence rests on more than mere noun learning, and requires mastery of grammatical constructs such as verb agreement (e.g., "The boy smiles at the man"), pluralization, and the use of passive sentence structure ("The car was driven by the woman"). Some research suggests that this fuller examination of language is a better predictor not only of future language, but also of future reading outcomes (NICHD, 2005).

We are also aware that language is characterized not only by the *products* of learning or the outcomes, but also by the *processes* of learning (Fisher, 1996; Hirsh-Pasek & Golinkoff, 1996; Hirsh-Pasek, Kochanoff, Newcombe, & De Villiers, 2005; Marcus, Vijayan, Bandi Rao, & Vishton, 1999; Saffran, Aslin, & Newport, 1996; Seymour, Roeper, & de Villiers, 2004). Processes, such as *fast mapping*, that help children connect a word and a referent with few exposures are hallmarks of language processing that are amenable to assessment. Indeed, there is also growing evidence in the literature that it is these early processes that predict later observable language milestones (Hurtado, Marchman, & Fernald, 2008; Tsao, Liu, & Kuhl, 2004). Process indicators might also be better predictors of success in learning than observable milestones because they tend to be less culturally and linguistically biased and less influenced by environmental variables.

Following norming, IRT item calibrations will again be recalculated, and any weaker items permanently removed from the item bank. Spanish versions of these instruments have also been developed and will be validated as part of the national norming study.

Data from the norming study will enable numerous examinations of the performance of these new instruments, as well as the assessment of hypotheses regarding the role of language acquisition relative to the other 45 constructs examined by the NIH Toolbox. We expect to find that reliability is poorest for emerging readers whose language acquisition appears to be the most inconsistent. In an attempt to further examine the relation between language attainment of children and their parents' education, we hope 1 day to assess the vocabulary of parent–child dyads. We would obtain language scores from children and their parents, as well as their respective levels of education. Vocabulary comprehension and reading decoding could be explored in relation not only to the other measures of cognition, but also to emotional health and sensory functioning as well. (Note: As of the date of publication the norming of the NIH Toolbox is complete. Norming results are available at www.nihtoolbox.org.)

REFERENCES

Benedict, R. (1997). *Brief Visuospatial Memory Test—Revised: Professional Manual.* Odessa, FL: Psychological Assessment Resources.

Brown, G. D. A. (1984). A frequency count of 190,000 words in the London-Lund Corpus of English Conversation. *Behavior Research Methods, Instruments, & Computers,* **16**, 502–532.

Burton, C. L., Strauss, E., Hultsch, D. F., & Hunter, M. A. (2006). Cognitive functioning and everyday problem solving in older adults. *Clinical Neuropsychologist,* **20**(3), 432–452.

Caplan, D., & Hildebrandt, N. (1988). *Disorders of syntactic comprehension.* Cambridge, MA: MIT Press.

Cattell, R. B. (1987). *Intelligence: Its structure, growth and action.* Amsterdam: Elsevier.

Dale, E., & O'Rourke, J. (1976). *The living word vocabulary: The words we know: A national vocabulary inventory.* Elgin, IL: Field Enterprises Educational Corp.; distributed exclusively by Dome.

Dickinson, D. K., Golinkoff, R. M., & Hirsh-Pasek, K. (2010). Speaking out for language: Why language is central to reading development. *Educational Researcher,* **39**(4), 305–310.

Dunn, L. M., & Dunn, D. M. (2007). *Peabody picture vocabulary test* (4th ed.). San Antonio, TX: Pearson.

Fenson, L., Dale, P. S., Reznick, J. S., Bates, E., Thal, D. J., & Pethick, S. J. (1994). Variability in early communicative development. *Monographs of the Society for Research in Child Development,* **59**(5), 1–173.

Fisher, C. (1996). Structural limits on verb mapping: The role of analogy in children's interpretations of sentences. *Cognitive Psychology,* **31**(1), 41–81.

Friederici, A. D., Rüschemeyer, S. A., Hahne, A., & Fiebach, C. J. (2003). The role of left inferior frontal and superior temporal cortex in sentence comprehension: Localizing syntactic and semantic processes. *Cerebral Cortex,* **13**(2), 170–177.

Gershon, R. C. (1988). *Index of words in the Johnson O'Connor Research Foundation, Inc. Vocabulary Item Bank.* New York: Johnson O'Connor Research Foundation Human Engineering Laboratory.

Gershon, R. C., Cella, D., Fox, N. A., Havlik, R. J., Hendrie, H. C., & Wagster, M. V. (2010). Assessment of neurological and behavioural function: The NIH Toolbox. *Lancet Neurology,* **9**(2), 138–139.

Gleason, J. B. (1997). *The development of language.* Boston: Allyn and Bacon.

Gleason, J. B., & Ratner, N. B. (2009). *The development of language* (7th ed.). Boston: Pearson/Allyn and Bacon.

Grober, E., & Sliwinski, M. (1991). Development and validation of a model for estimating premorbid verbal intelligence in the elderly. *Journal of Clinical and Experimental Neuropsychology,* **13**(6), 933–949.

Hirsch, C., & Wexler, K. (2007). The late acquisition of raising: What children seem to think about seem. In W. D. Davies & S. Dubinsky (Eds.), *New horizons in the analysis of control and raising* (pp. 35–70). New York: Springer.

Hirsh-Pasek, K., & Golinkoff, R. M. (1996). *The origins of grammar: Evidence from early language comprehension.* Cambridge, MA: MIT Press.

Hirsh-Pasek, K., Kochanoff, A. T., Newcombe, N., & De Villiers, J. (2005). Using scientific knowledge to inform preschool assessment: Making the case for empirical validity. *Society for Research in Child Development Social Policy Report,* **19**(1), 3–19.

Hurtado, N., Marchman, V. A., & Fernald, A. (2008). Does input influence uptake? Links between maternal talk, processing speed and vocabulary size in spanish-learning children. *Developmental Science*, **11**(6), 31.

Kastner, J. W., May, W., & Hildman, L. (2001). Relationship between language skills and academic achievement in first grade. *Perceptual and Motor Skills*, **92**(2), 381–390.

Kucera, H., & Francis, W. N. (1967). *Computational analysis of present-day American English*. Providence: Brown University Press.

Kuhl, P., & Rivera-Gaxiola, M. (2008). Neural substrates of language acquisition. *Annual Review of Neuroscience*, **31**, 511–534.

Kuhl, P. K. (2004). Early language acquisition: Cracking the speech code. *Nature Reviews Neuroscience*, **5**(11), 831–843.

Linacre, J. M. (2005). *A user's guide to WINSTEPS/MINISTEP: Rasch-model computer programs*. Chicago, IL: Winsteps.

Manly, J. J., Byrd, D. A., Touradji, P., & Stern, Y. (2004). Acculturation, reading level, and neuropsychological test performance among african american elders. *Applied Neuropsychology*, **11**(1), 37–46.

Manly, J. J., Jacobs, D. M., Sano, M., Bell, K., Merchant, C. A., Small, S. A., et al. (1999). Effect of literacy on neuropsychological test performance in nondemented, education-matched elders. *Journal of the International Neuropsychological Society*, **5**(3), 191–202.

Marcus, G. F., Vijayan, S., Bandi Rao, S., & Vishton, P. M. (1999). Rule learning by seven-month-old infants. *Science*, **283**(5398), 77–80.

Meisinger, E. B., Bloom, J. S., & Hynd, G. W. (2010). Reading fluency: Implications for the assessment of children with reading disabilities. *Annals of Dyslexia*, **60**(1), 1–17.

Mogilner, A. (1992). *Children's writer's word book*. Cincinnati, OH: Writer's Digest Books.

National Early Literacy Panel, & National Center for Family Literacy. (2008). Developing early literacy report of the National Early Literacy Panel, from http://purl.access.gpo.gov/GPO/LPS108121

National Reading Panel, & National Institute of Child Health and Human Development. (2000). *National Reading Panel: Teaching children to read: An evidence-based assessment of the scientific research literature on reading and its implications for reading instruction: Reports of the subgroups*. Washington, DC: National Institute of Child Health and Human Development, National Institutes of Health.

National Research Council Committee on the Prevention of Reading Difficulties in Young Children, Snow, C. E., Burns, M. S., Griffin, P., & National Research Council Commission on Behavioral Social Sciences Education. (2002). *Preventing reading difficulties in young children: Intellectual property in the information age* (8th ed.). Washington, DC: National Academies Press.

NICHD Early Child Care Research Network. (2005). Pathways to reading: The role of oral language in the transition to reading. *Developmental Psychology*, **41**(2), 428–442.

Pinker, S. (2000). *The language instinct: How the mind creates language*. New York: Perennial Classics.

Price, C. J. (1998). The functional anatomy of word comprehension and production. *Trends in Cognitive Sciences*, **2**(8), 281–287.

Price, C. J. (2000). The anatomy of language: Contributions from functional neuroimaging. *Journal of Anatomy*, **197**(3), 335–359.

Rapcsak, S. Z., Henry, M. L., Teague, S. L., Carnahan, S. D., & Beeson, P. M. (2007). Do dual-route models accurately predict reading and spelling performance in individuals with acquired alexia and agraphia? *Neuropsychologia*, 45(11), 2519–2524.

Rasch, G. (1960). *Probabilistic models for some intelligence and attainment tests.* Copenhagen: Dansmarks Paedagogiske Institut.

Rey, A. (1958). *L'Examen clinique en psychologie.* Paris: Press Universitaire de France.

Saffran, J. R., Aslin, R. N., & Newport, E. L. (1996). Statistical learning by 8-month-old infants. *Science*, 274(5294), 1926–1928.

Schmidt, F. L., & Hunter, J. (2004). General mental ability in the world of work: Occupational attainment and job performance. *Journal of Personality and Social Psychology*, 86(1), 162–173. doi: 10.1037/0022-3514.86.1.162

Seymour, H. N., Roeper, T., & de Villiers, J. G. (2004). Conclusions, future directions, and implications for remediation. *Seminars in Speech and Language*, 25(1), 113–115.

Sternberg, R. J. (2004). Intelligence in humans. In S. Charles (Ed.), *Encyclopedia of Applied Psychology* (pp. 321–328). New York: Elsevier.

Tsao, F.-M., Liu, H.-M., & Kuhl, P. K. (2004). Speech perception in infancy predicts language development in the second year of life: A longitudinal study. *Child Development*, 75(4), 1067–1084.

University of Western Australia School of Psychology. (2011). MRC Psycholinguistic Database Retrieved May 5, 2011, from http://www.psy.uwa.edu.au/mrcdatabase/uwa_mrc.htm

Wilkinson, G. S., & Robertson, G. J. (2006). *WRAT 4: Wide range achievement test professional manual.* Lutz, FL: Psychological Assessment Resources.

Wolf, M. S., Gazmararian, J. A., & Baker, D. W. (2005). Health literacy and functional health status among older adults. *Archives of Internal Medicine*, 165(17), 1946–1952.

Ziegler, J. C., Castel, C., Pech-Georgel, C., George, F., Alario, F. X., & Perry, C. (2008). Developmental dyslexia and the dual route model of reading: Simulating individual differences and subtypes. *Cognition*, 107(1), 151–178.

V. NIH TOOLBOX COGNITION BATTERY (CB): MEASURING WORKING MEMORY

David S. Tulsky, Noelle E. Carlozzi, Nicolas Chevalier, Kimberly A. Espy, Jennifer L. Beaumont, and Dan Mungas

ABSTRACT This chapter focuses on the NIH Toolbox List Sorting Working Memory Test, which was developed to assess processing speed within the NIH Toolbox Cognition Battery (CB). This test is a sequencing task requiring children and adults to process stimuli (presented both visually and auditorily) and sequence the stimuli according to size. We describe the development of the NIH Toolbox List Sorting Working Memory Test, highlighting its utility in children. We examine descriptive data, test–retest reliability, and convergent and discriminant validity. Results indicated that List Sorting performance was positively correlated with age indicating that performance on the task improved throughout childhood and early adolescence. Further, test–retest reliability coefficients were high and there was support for both convergent and discriminant validity. These data suggest that the NIH Toolbox List Sorting Working Memory Test is reliable and shows evidence of construct validity.

In this chapter, we discuss the development of the Toolbox List Sorting Working Memory Test, a new measure of working memory.

Subdomain Definition

Working memory is probably one of the most widely studied constructs in psychology due to its prominent role in complex cognitive tasks and daily activities (e.g., mental arithmetic and reading). It is a capacity-limited system devoted to holding information in mind over brief periods of time, typically while manipulating it for ongoing activity. Given the importance of this construct, a wide number of tasks have been designed to assess it. In young children, working memory tasks tend to focus on actively maintaining information over brief intervals in the face of interference. From preschool

---

Corresponding author: David S. Tulsky, North Campus Research Complex, 2800 Plymouth Road, Building NCRC B520, Office 3210, Ann Arbor, MI 48109-2800, email: dtulsky@med.umich.edu

age on, most tasks either require retaining and reorganizing items before recalling them (e.g., backward digit span task), or completing some processing activity in between presentations of the to-be-recalled items (e.g., listening span task). Such tasks tap into both information processing and storage, and yield a working memory span measure that corresponds to the maximal amount of accurately recalled information.

The cognitive structure of working memory is actively debated. Baddeley and Hitch's (1974) tripartite model is one of the most influential models of working memory. It identifies two domain-specific components, the *phonological loop* and *visuospatial sketchpad* (devoted to temporary storage of verbal and visuospatial information, respectively), and a domain-general component, the *central executive* (responsible for filtering out irrelevant information, integrating the information held in the other two components and in long-term memory and supervising this processing). A fourth component—the *episodic buffer*—was subsequently added as the storage locus for integrated information (Baddeley, 2000). The central executive also is a main component of Cowan's (2005) model, which posits working memory as the activated element of long-term memory, wherein the most strongly activated information—the *focus of attention*—receives direct attention from the central executive. Because resources of the central executive are limited, the degree of control dilutes as the amount of information increases in the focus of attention (whose capacity is limited to three to four items). Building on the proposal of two levels of activation in working memory, Unsworth and Engle (2007) argued that, when information no longer receives attention, it leaves the focus of attention and must subsequently be retrieved from the activated long-term memory using context cues. Both active maintenance in the focus of attention and retrieval processes from activated long-term memory allegedly tax the central executive and contribute to working memory capacity. Despite structural differences across theoretical models (Cowan, 2005; Engle, Kane, & Tuholski, 1999; Miyake & Shah, 1999), all models identify temporary storage and control components, as illustrated by Engle et al.'s (1999) formula, working memory = short-term memory + controlled attention.

Working memory encompasses short-term memory (i.e., temporary storage of information, irrespective of processing demands) and shares its properties. In particular, information in working memory is short-lived and susceptible to the interference created by goal-irrelevant information unless it is shielded and/or actively maintained through attention control. Given this prominent role of attention control, working memory also is intermingled with the construct of executive function, that is, the set of cognitive processes that support goal-oriented thought and action. Executive processes are considered to comprise inhibiting irrelevant information, switching task sets, updating working memory content, and maintaining information in an active state (e.g., Garon, Bryson, & Smith, 2008; Miyake et al., 2000; Munakata, 2001; Zelazo et al., Chapter 2, this volume). Therefore, executive function can be viewed as the processes by which the central executive component operates. In the developmental literature, working memory is often conceived as a subset of executive functions, but in such case, working memory generally refers to the active maintenance process (instead of the whole construct of working memory). Consistently, tasks assessing working memory and executive functions load onto a single latent factor in children under 7 years of age, lending support to substantial shared variation between the two constructs (Shing, Lindenberger, Diamond, Li, & Davidson, 2010; Wiebe, Espy, & Charak, 2008; Wiebe et al., 2011).

Importance During Childhood

Working memory development has a tremendous impact on children's cognition as it is associated with academic achievement, including mathematic skills and reading skills (e.g., Bull & Scerif, 2001; Nevo & Breznitz, 2011). Temporary maintenance and manipulation of information is required during learning episodes in the classroom as these often require remembering lengthy instructions. Thus, low working memory capacity puts children at risk for poor academic progress (Alloway & Gathercole, 2006; Alloway, Gathercole, Kirkwood, & Elliott, 2009). In addition, working memory deficits, especially in verbal short-term memory, have been associated with reading difficulties and developmental dyslexia (e.g., Gathercole, Alloway, Willis, & Adams, 2006; Smith-Spark & Fisk, 2007). Working memory deficits also have been reported in a variety of developmental disorders including Attention Deficit/ Hyperactivity Disorder (e.g., Willcutt, Doyle, Nigg, Faraone, & Pennington, 2005), specific language impairment (e.g., Briscoe & Rankin, 2009), and autism (e.g., Williams, Goldstein, & Minshew, 2006), as well as prematurity (e.g., Vicari, Caravale, Carlesimo, Casadei, & Allemand, 2004), traumatic brain injury (e.g., Levin et al., 2004), and childhood cancer (Dennis et al., 1991). Although individual differences in working memory capacity are relatively stable over time, recent evidence suggests that working memory capacity can be effectively improved through intervention programs during childhood (Holmes, Gathercole, & Dunning, 2009; Thorell, Lindqvist, Bergman Nutley, Bohlin, & Klingberg, 2009). Such evidence opens up avenues to remediate low working memory capacity in children and enhance academic outcome, and therefore reinforces the need for precise identification of at-risk children through adequate assessment of working memory during childhood.

Relations of Domain With Brain Function

In adults and older children, working memory task performance is sustained by a distributed fronto-parietal network that includes parietal cortex ventro- and dorso-lateral prefrontal cortex (Bunge, Klingberg, Jacobsen, & Gabrieli, 2000; Kwon, Reiss, & Menon, 2002; Wager & Smith, 2003). Some studies additionally report involvement of the anterior cingulate cortex, basal ganglia (especially, the striatum), medial temporal cortex, and cerebellum (Chein, Moore, & Conway, 2011; McNab & Klingberg, 2008; O'Hare, Lu, Houston, Bookheimer, & Sowell, 2008; Osaka et al., 2004). Consistent with the role of prefrontal regions in executive function (e.g., Casey, Galvan, & Hare, 2005), evidence suggests that these regions and basal ganglia act as a selective gating mechanism that controls the information accessing working memory and maintained in parietal regions (McNab & Klingberg, 2008; Postle, 2006). Further evidence comes from findings that the nature of the task items influence activation in the parietal lobe (left-lateralized for verbal items, right-lateralized for visuospatial items; Thomason et al., 2009), but not in prefrontal regions (Wager & Smith, 2003). Although prefrontal regions may support domain-general processes, dorsal prefrontal regions may be especially involved in information manipulation whereas ventral prefrontal regions may more strongly relate to active maintenance of the information stored in posterior regions (D'Esposito, Postle, Ballard, & Lease, 1999; Wager & Smith, 2003).

Working memory capacity develops on a protracted course. As early as 6 months of age, infants are able to retain information over brief intervals in spite of distraction (Reznick, Morrow, Goldman, & Snyder, 2004). Working-memory capacity then steadily improves through late adolescence (Gathercole, Pickering, Ambridge, & Wearing, 2004; McAuley & White, 2011). On average, a preschooler's working memory span triples by early adulthood (Dempster, 1981), although at each age span length varies as a function of context-specific demands (Conlin, Gathercole, & Adams, 2005). The tripartite structure of working memory (verbal and visuospatial short-term stores along with a control entity) is observable from age 4 years on, suggesting that little structural change occurs after that age, although the relation between visuospatial information storage and executive function seems stronger between ages 4 and 6 years than later in childhood (Alloway, Gathercole, & Pickering, 2006; Gathercole et al., 2004). However, visuospatial information may heavily draw upon executive function in adulthood as well (Miyake, Friedman, Rettinger, Shah, & Hegarty, 2001). Consistent with evidence of constant working memory structure across ages, children recruit the same fronto-parietal network while performing working memory tasks as do adults (e.g., Nelson et al., 2000). With age, however, activation in these regions becomes stronger and more focal, and as children get older, working memory involves other regions such as the cerebellum. This is also common in adults as working-memory demands increase (Geier, Garver, Terwilliger, & Luna, 2009; Kwon et al., 2002; Thomason et al., 2009).

Developmental change in working memory is driven by age-related increase in both temporary storage capacity and control efficiency (see Cowan, 2010; Gathercole et al., 2004), the latter probably being related to improvement in executive function (e.g., Best, Miller, & Jones, 2009; Carlson, 2005). In addition to such quantitative improvements, working memory development also results from change in strategy use over age (e.g., Barrouillet & Camos, 2011). Rehearsal of verbal information is an especially efficient strategy whose corresponding neural circuit (including Broca's area, premotor cortex, and inferior parietal areas) is part of the fronto-parietal network associated with working memory (e.g., Kwon et al., 2002). Yet, only around age 7 years do children start verbally rehearsing information spontaneously (see Gathercole & Hitch, 1993). Similarly, with age, children become increasingly prone to recode visuospatial information into a phonological format so that it can be rehearsed more easily (Hitch & Halliday, 1983).

Processing speed is another important factor to consider. Indeed, increase in processing speed has been shown to account for up to 75% of the variance in working memory improvement with age (Fry & Hale, 2000; Kail & Hall, 2001; McAuley & White, 2011; Nettelbeck & Burns, 2010). According to cascade theory (Fry & Hale, 1996), age-related improvement in processing speed drives changes in working memory which, in turn, lead to increasing fluid intelligence (see also Case, 1987). There are at least two potential reasons why working memory span increases with processing speed. First, faster processing speed may speed up the rate of verbal rehearsal, hence improving information maintenance (Fry & Hale, 2000). Second, higher processing speed may accelerate information manipulation and therefore leave extra time when attention can be allocated to information maintenance (Barrouillet, Bernardin, & Camos, 2004; Towse, Hitch, & Hutton, 1998). Prominent as the role of processing speed may be, part of working memory change occurs independently of this skill (McAuley & White, 2011).

NIH Toolbox CB Measurement

Development of the Toolbox List Sorting Working Memory Test

The Toolbox List Sorting Working Memory Test is a sequencing task requiring children and adults to sort information and sequence it. Items are presented both visually and auditorily. The participants (either children or adults) are presented with a series of illustrated pictures, each depicting an item (e.g., an animal) on the computer, along with their auditory names. Each item is displayed for 2 sec. Participants are instructed to remember the stimuli but to repeat them verbally to the examiner in order of size, from smallest to largest. The number of objects in a series increase on successive items thereby taxing the working memory system when longer sequences

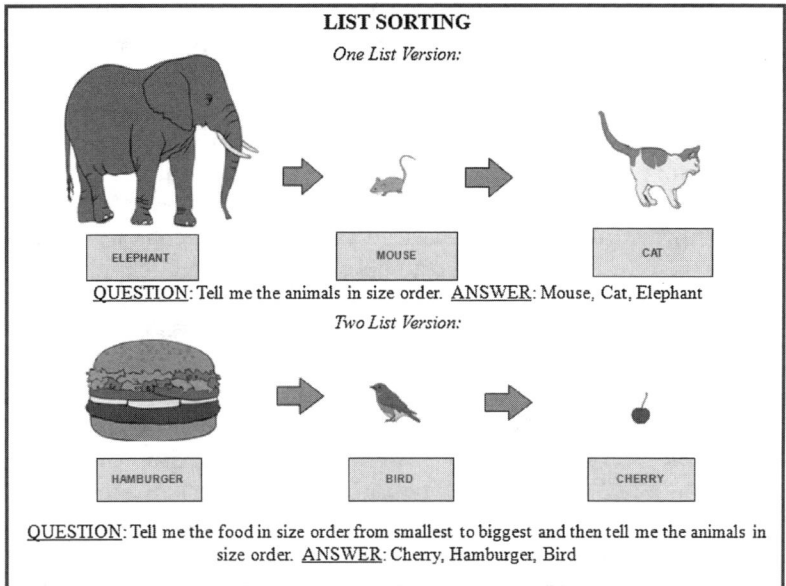

FIGURE 9.—Examples of one-list and two-list list sorting task.
Note. 1-List List Sorting requires participants to sequence items according to a single category, whereas 2-List List Sorting requires sequencing that involves an alternation between two different categories. For both 1- and 2-List List Sorting, each picture was displayed for 2 sec.

need to be remembered. Furthermore, the task starts with a "1-list" version where the children have to sequence one type of stimuli (e.g., "animals" or "food") according to size order and then switch to a "2-list" version where two types of stimuli have to be sequenced, each in size order. In the 2-list version, the working memory load is increased substantially as the stimuli are presented from two categories (animals and food) and the participant has to track and organize stimuli from both categories and report by size the items from one category (i.e., animals) and then the other category by size (i.e., food). It is this "dual" tracking and processing information that increases the working memory load of the task. See Figure 9 for an example of 1-List and 2-List items.

Other sequencing tasks include the Letter Number Sequencing Test (Gold, Carpenter, Randolph, Goldberg, & Weinberger, 1997) that was incorporated into the Wechsler Intelligence Scales (WAIS-III, WAIS-IV, and WISC-IV) (Tulsky, Saklofske, & Zhu, 2003; Wechsler, 1997, 2003, 2008) and the Spanish and English Neuropsychological Assessment Scales (SENAS) Working Memory task (Crane et al., 2008; Mungas, Reed, Tomaszewski Farias, & DeCarli, 2005). The Toolbox List Sorting Working Memory Test that we have developed is modeled after the SENAS, which is an auditory working memory test; stimuli are presented both visually (object) and auditorily (corresponding word) in an attempt to make the task easier and more relevant to children. The earliest versions of the Toolbox List Sorting Working Memory Test provided children with multiple opportunities for practice (prior to the administration of actual test items). Children were given two practice items involve sequencing of toy animals, followed by computerized items presenting all items on the screen simultaneously, followed by practice items involving individual administration of each item in the series.

Preparing the Toolbox List Sorting Working Memory Test for Children

Most working memory tests are developed using one modality, either visual or auditory, and the tests are often used to evaluate cognition the specific subsystems of this cognitive process (e.g., visuospatial sketchpad, phenomenological loop). In the case of the Toolbox, the distinction between visual and auditory working memory was less important than a more general assessment of cognitive functioning over the lifespan, and the test development team had visual images drawn to accompany auditory presentation of the stimuli. The logic was that the visual images would enhance the usability of the task for children. Three preliminary studies were conducted to adapt the List Sorting task for pediatric use and ensure that the task is relevant to children.

For the first pilot study, ten 3 year olds were recruited from a local nursery school. The goal of this study was to examine task feasibility of list sorting. Children were shown the visual pictures of the objects and asked to repeat what they had seen except reorder them according to size, smallest to largest. The children received three practice items before the test began. We examined the range of scores on test items for our participants to determine test feasibility. We also examined performance on practice items to determine if children as young as 3 years of age were able to understand the basic tenets of this task; children were given up to three training trials on each item, prior to moving on to the next item. Three-year-olds scores ranged from 0 to 5 on the 1-list, and 0 to 3 on the 2-list. Further, all children were able to complete all of the practice items within the three training trials. These results suggested that children as young as 3 years of age were able to understand the basic concepts of the task. In general, children were able to sequence items in size order. From these data, we revised the task, increasing the number of items on both the 1-list and 2-list to increase the range of scores.

In the second pilot study, we administered the revised version of List Sorting to 47 children ages 3–6 years. Twenty-two participants completed a retest within 2 weeks. We examined the range, mean, standard deviation, and test–retest reliability to determine task feasibility. Results indicated that children as young as 3 years of age could complete the initial items on the

Toolbox List Sorting Working Memory Test. For the 1-list total score, the range of scores for 3–6 year olds was 0–16 with an average score of 6.67 ($SD = 4.42$). Performance was lower for the 2-list component of the test as the range was 0–10 with an average score of 3.4 ($SD = 2.33$), which is expected given that the 2-list task is more challenging. Test–retest reliability coefficients were $r = .85$ and $r = .86$, respectively, for both the 1-list and 2-list task, indicating that the performance was highly reliable. These pilot data indicated that children as young as 3 years of age were able to sequence items in size order. The results also helped us modify the List Sorting task further as we added some easier items to further increase the range of scores. We also combined scores on the 1- and 2-list tasks to increase the range and variability of scores on this task.

In the third ("prevalidation") pilot study, we administered the Toolbox List Sorting Working Memory Test to three groups of children ages 3–4 years ($n = 35$), 5–7 ($n = 26$), and 8–14 years ($n = 28$). The goal was to fully examine the descriptive statistics of the Toolbox List Sorting Working Memory Test across different age bands along with a closer examination of the test–retest reliability of the test. Our results indicated that cognitive abilities across childhood improve. Performance on the combined 1-list and 2-list score in the 3- to 4-year-old children ranged from 5 to 28 with an average score of 18.3 ($SD = 6.5$). Performance in the 5- to 7-year-old group ranged from 9 to 37 with a mean of 28.4 ($SD = 5.5$). Finally, performance in the 8- to 14-year-old group ranged from 32 to 48 with a mean of 40.6 ($SD = 4.5$). Test–retest reliability was highest in the youngest group ($r = .90$), $r = .79$ in the 5–7 year olds, and $r = .74$ in the 8- to 14-year-old group. The results again indicated that most children were able to understand the basic concepts of List Sorting. Further, test–retest reliability was best for the youngest ages.

The testing also allowed us to examine item difficulty and remove redundancy from the test so that we could streamline administration, shorten the length of the task, and drop poor performing items. The findings provided justification for removing a portion of practice items, and creating discontinuation rules for children that were unable to answer all practice items correctly (they would not be administered the test). The validation version of this test was prepared and the next section discusses the results of the validation study for children ages 3–15 years. Data from adults will be published separately so that each population can be addressed in greater depth.

METHOD

Participants

The participants in the validation study are described in detail in Weintraub et al. (Chapter 1, this volume; Table 3). Nine children (all age 6 and younger) failed the practice items or otherwise did not successfully complete the task for reasons such as lack of attention or alertness or general noncompliance.

Measures

Participants were tested with the Toolbox List Sorting Working Memory Test as well as several additional tasks to provide convergent (the Developmental Neuropsychological Assessment, 2nd Edition Sentence Repetition subtest; the Wechsler Intelligence Scale for Children, 4th Edition Letter-Number Sequencing subtest) and discriminant validity (the Peabody Picture Vocabulary Test, 4th Edition, the Delis–Kaplan Executive Function System Color-Word Test, and the Wisconsin Card Sorting Test-64 Card Version).

The Toolbox List Sorting Working Memory Test

In this task, a list of stimuli is presented both visually (picture) and auditorily (recording of a one-word description of the stimulus) on a computer monitor, one at a time at a rate of 2 sec per stimulus, and participants are required to repeat all of the stimuli back to the examiner in order of increasing real-world size, from smallest to largest. On practice trials, participants are required to reorder and repeat the items in a 2-item list (e.g., List: pumpkin, lemon; Correct answer: "Lemon, pumpkin"), followed by a 3-item list.

In the first phase of the test (i.e., the 1-List phase), participants are first shown a list with 2 items drawn from a single category (i.e., food). If participants are correct on this 2-item list, the number of items in the list presented on the next trial increases by one item, up to a total of 7 items per list (i.e., list length ranges from a 2-item list to a 7-item list, for a total of six levels of list length). If participants err on a trial at a given list length, they receive another trial with the same number of items in the list; if they err on that trial, this phase of the test is discontinued. That is, the 1-List phase of the test is discontinued when two trials of the same list length are failed.

Following the 1-List phase, all participants proceed to the second phase of the test (the 2-List phase), in which they see lists of items drawn from two different categories (i.e., food and animals). Participants are instructed to reorder and repeat the stimuli first from one category, then the other, in order of size within each category. Lists in the 2-List phase start with a 2-item list and increase in number of items in the same way as in the 1-List phase (i.e., from a 2-item list to a 7-item list, for a total of six levels of list length).

For both phases, for each list length, participants receive a score of 2 points if they are correct on the first trial. A second trial at a given list length is only administered when participants fail the first trial. Participants receive a score of 1 point only for a given list length if they fail the first trial at that list length but pass the second trial. Test scores consist of combined total trials correct on the 1-List and 2-List phases of the task. The test takes approximately 10 min to administer.

Convergent Validity

The Developmental Neuropsychological Assessment, 2nd Edition Sentence Repetition (NEPSY-II Sentence Repetition; Korkman, Kirk, & Kemp, 2007) involves an examiner reading a series of sentences of increasing complexity and length. The participant is required to recall each sentence after each is presented. Participants ages 3–6 years completed this measure. For analysis we used the Sentence Repetition Total Score.

For children ages 8–15 years, the measure of convergent validity was the Wechsler Intelligence Scale for Children, 4th Edition (WISC-IV) Letter-Number Sequencing (Wechsler, 2008). In this test, participants are presented with a mixed list of numbers and letters, and their task is to repeat the list by saying the numbers first in ascending order and then the letters in alphabetical order. Scores reflect the number of correct responses (maximum 30 points), with higher scores indicating better performance.

Discriminant Validity

The Peabody Picture Vocabulary Test, 4th Edition (PPVT-IV; Dunn & Dunn, 2007) provides a measure of receptive vocabulary and word retrieval. Examinees are asked to identify which of four pictures reflects a specific word. Scores are based on the number correct (maximum 228). Participants ages 3–15 years completed this measure.

The Delis–Kaplan Executive Function System Color-Word test (D-KEFS Color-Word; Delis, Kaplan, & Kramer, 2001) is based on the Stroop procedure and taps the participants' ability to inhibit overlearned verbal responses. Specifically, the participant is timed during his or her (1) naming of color patches; (2) reading basic color words printed in black ink; and (3) naming the color of the ink in which color words are printed. In the last condition, the colors of the ink and the printed color words differ from each other. Participants ages 8–15 years completed this measure. For this study, we examined scores on the Color-Word interference score.

The Wisconsin Card Sorting Test-64 Card Version (WCST-64; Kongs, Thompson, Iverson, & Heaton, 2000) is a shortened, 64-card version of the Wisconsin Card Sorting Test, which assesses the ability to shift sets using visual stimuli that are easily verbally mediated. It requires participants to sort pictured cards into piles according to changing rules. Successful completion of the test relies on having a number of intact cognitive functions including attention, working memory, and visual processing. Participants ages 8–15 years completed this measure. We examined perseverative errors for this study.

Data Analysis

This study examines associations of the Toolbox List Sorting Working Memory Test scores with age, test–retest reliability, and convergent and discriminant validity. Pearson correlation coefficients between age and Toolbox List Sorting Working Memory Test performance were calculated to describe the developmental-related associations for each measure. Intraclass correlation coefficients (*ICC*) were calculated to evaluate test–retest reliability and convergent and discriminant validity. Convergent validity was assessed with correlations between the Toolbox List Sorting Working Memory Test and established measures of the same construct (i.e., NEPSY-II Sentence Completion and WISC-IV Letter Number Sequencing); evidence of discriminant validity consisted of lower correlations with selected validation measures of *different* cognitive constructs: receptive vocabulary (PPVT-IV) and executive function (DKEFS Color-Word and WCST).

RESULTS

Age Effects

Figure 10 provides a graphic presentation of performance on the Toolbox List Sorting Working Memory Test from ages 3 to 15 years. Across these ages, age was related to performance on the test ($df = 199$, $r = .77$, $p < .0001$), and a quadratic model provided the best fit of the data, with

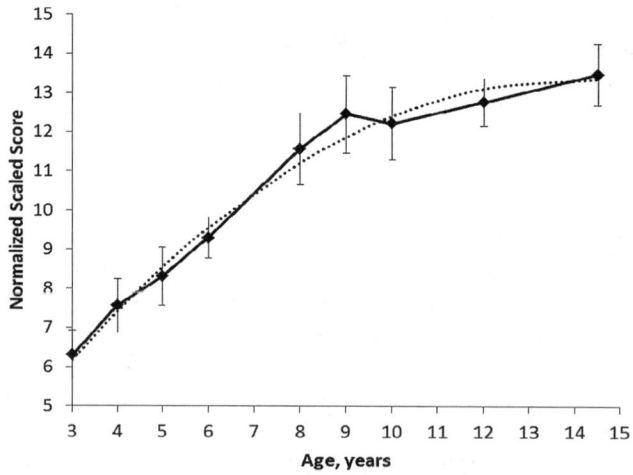

FIGURE 10.—Normalized scaled scores on the Toolbox List Sorting Working Memory Test across age groups. Error bars are ±2 standard errors. Best-fitting polynomial curve is also shown (see text).

$R^2 = .66$. Positive associations between age and test performance were also seen for ages 3–6 years ($df = 111$, $r = .52$, $p < .0001$) and for ages 8–15 years ($df = 86$, $r = .33$, $p = .002$). Pairwise comparisons between age groups are reported in Appendix A.

Test–Retest Reliability

Overall *ICC* for the Toolbox List Sorting Working Memory Test (ages 3–15 years) was .86 (95% CI = .78, .91), which was higher than the test–retest reliability for NEPSY-II Sentence Repetition for ages 3–6 years ($ICC = .80$, 95% CI = .65, .89), and WISC-IV Letter Number Sequencing for ages 8–15 years ($ICC = .80$, 95% CI = .52, .87).

Effect of Repeated Testing

Practice effects were computed as the difference between test and retest normalized scaled scores, with significance of the effect being tested with t tests for dependent means. For the total child group (ages 3–15 years, $n = 66$), the Toolbox List Sorting Working Memory Test showed no practice effect over an average 2-week test–retest interval: *mean practice effect* = 0.15, $SD = 1.68$, $t(65) = .72$, $p = .48$.

Construct Validity

Table 10 shows results for convergent and discriminant validity. Correlations for convergent validity were .57 for both ages 3–6 years and 8–

TABLE 10

PEARSON CORRELATIONS BETWEEN THE TOOLBOX LIST SORTING WORKING MEMORY TEST AND CONVERGENT AND DISCRIMINANT VALIDATION MEASURES

	Ages 3–6 years		Age 8–15 years	
	df	r	df	r
Convergent validity measures				
NEPSY-II Sentence Completion	107	.57	—	—
WISC-IV Letter-Number Sequencing	—	—	83	.57
Discriminant validity measures				
PPVT-IV	110	.63	85	.45
D-KEFS Color-Word Interference	—	—	84	.45
WCST-64 Perseverative Errors	—	—	85	.42

Note. r, Pearson's Correlation Coefficient; NEPSY-II, Developmental Neuropsychological Assessment Battery, 2nd Edition; WISC-IV, Wechsler Intelligence Scale for Children, 4th Edition; PPVT-IV, Peabody Picture Vocabulary Test-4th Edition; Unadjusted scaled scores; D-KEFS, Delis–Kaplan Executive Function System; WCST-64, Wisconsin Card Sorting Test-64 Card version. © 2006–2012 National Institutes of Health and Northwestern University.
All $ps \leq .0001$.

15 years (all $p \leq .0001$), suggesting that the List Sorting, NEPSY-II Sentence Completion (3–6 years), and WISC-IV Letter Number Sequencing (8–15 years) tasks tap a similar construct, and have adequate convergent validity. The correlations with the discriminant validity measure (the PPVT-IV/receptive vocabulary) were $r = .63$ ($df = 110$, $p < .0001$) in the younger children and $r = .45$ ($df = 85$, $p < .0001$) in the older children indicating an overlap with this construct. Discriminant correlations did not differ significantly from the corresponding convergent correlations.

DISCUSSION

In this chapter we described the development and validation of a new measure of working memory, the Toolbox List Sorting Working Memory Test, with specific emphasis on how this measure was developed and adapted for use in a pediatric population. Stimuli were prepared in an auditory and visual modality so that the test would yield a general working memory score (independent of modality) and would not distinguish between specific structural working memory components like the phonological loop or visuospatial sketchpad.

As noted above, most children were able to understand the basic sequencing tenets of List Sorting. Toolbox List Sorting Working Memory Test performance was correlated with age. That is, performance on the task improved throughout childhood and early adolescence. This is consistent with the anticipated developmental trajectory of working memory (Dempster, 1981; Gathercole et al., 2004; McAuley & White, 2011). Further, test–retest reliability was relatively high when computed across the entire 3- to 15-year age range.

In addition to reliability, the Toolbox List Sorting Working Memory Test also showed adequate convergent validity. Correlation coefficients were in the moderately high range when compared with criteria measures purported to measure working memory. Further, correlations with receptive vocabulary were moderate for the 3- to 6-year-old group showing that, for this younger group, the working memory task is correlated with verbal functioning. This likely represents general intelligence in the youngest children where specific domains of cognitive functioning are less defined (see Mungas et al., Chapter 7, this volume). The moderate correlations with traditional measures of executive function, as well as verbal functioning, in the 8–15 year olds also demonstrate that the working memory task is correlated with measures of general functioning, however, the correlations are somewhat lower than that with other working memory tasks (which suggest that the Toolbox List Sorting Working Memory Test has adequate convergent and discriminant validity).

In addition to our findings, it is also important to review some of the limitations of this study. First, the small sample sizes utilized within age bands make it difficult to evaluate test–retest correlations within age subgroups. This aspect of evaluation of the instrument will be remedied in the next phase of the task. Further, because stimuli for the Toolbox List Sorting Working Memory Test utilized both auditory and visual images, we are not able to distinguish between the specific components of the phonological loop or visuospatial sketchpad (Baddeley & Hitch, 1974).

Regardless of these limitations, the Toolbox List Sorting Working Memory Test presents a number of strengths. First, it is child-friendly and engaging, and it is short and easy to administer. Further, it is reliable and has demonstrated high content validity. It also requires size-order sequencing of both 1- and 2-category trials, which ensures that processing demands remain challenging throughout the lifespan (i.e., into adulthood). This is especially important given that other common measures of working memory (e.g., backward digit span tasks) are not as challenging for adults as they are for children. This fact implies that such tasks are appropriate measures of working memory in childhood, but not in adulthood (where the task reflects short-term memory rather than working memory; St. Clair-Thompson, 2010).

Following norming of the Toolbox List Sorting Working Memory Test future studies will be employed to examine the sensitivity of the Toolbox List Sorting Working Memory Test to neurological insult (e.g., traumatic brain injury). Ultimately, the Toolbox List Sorting Working Memory Test promises to provide a measure of working memory that is useful across the lifespan.

REFERENCES

Alloway, T. P., & Gathercole, S. E. (2006). How does working memory work in the classroom? *Educational Research and Reviews*, **1**, 134–139.

Alloway, T. P., Gathercole, S. E., Kirkwood, H., & Elliott, J. (2009). The cognitive and behavioral characteristics of children with low working memory. *Child Development*, **80**(2), 606–621.

Alloway, T. P., Gathercole, S. E., & Pickering, S. J. (2006). Verbal and visuospatial short-term and working memory in children: Are they separable? *Child Development*, **77**(6), 1698–1716.

Baddeley, A. (2000). The episodic buffer: A new component of working memory? *Trends in Cognitive Science*, **4**(11), 417–423.

Baddeley, A. D., & Hitch, G. J. (1974). *Working memory* (Vol. 8). New York: Academic Press.

Barrouillet, P., Bernardin, S., & Camos, V. (2004). Time constraints and resource sharing in adults' working memory spans. *Journal of Experimental Psychology: General*, **133**(1), 83–100.

Barrouillet, P., & Camos, V. (2011). Developmental change in working memory strategies: From passive maintenance to active refreshing. *Developmental Psychology*, **47**, 898–904.

Best, J. R., Miller, P. H., & Jones, L. L. (2009). Executive functions after age 5: Changes and correlates. *Developmental Review*, **29**(3), 180–200.

Briscoe, J., & Rankin, P. M. (2009). Exploration of a "double-jeopardy" hypothesis within working memory profiles for children with specific language impairment. *International Journal of Language & Communication Disorders*, **44**(2), 236–250.

Bull, R., & Scerif, G. (2001). Executive functioning as a predictor of children's mathematics ability: Inhibition, switching, and working memory. *Developmental Neuropsychology*, **19**(3), 273–293.

Bunge, S. A., Klingberg, T., Jacobsen, R. B., & Gabrieli, J. D. E. (2000). A resource model of the neural basis of executive working memory. *Proceedings of the National Academy of Sciences of the United States of America*, **97**(7), 3573–3578.

Carlson, S. A. (2005). Developmentally sensitive measures of executive function in preschool children. *Developmental Neuropsychology*, **28**(2), 595–616.

Case, R. (1987). The structure and process of intellectual development. *International Journal of Psychology*, **22**, 571–607.

Casey, B. J., Galvan, A., & Hare, T. A. (2005). Changes in cerebral functional organization during cognitive development. *Current Opinion in Neurobiology*, **15**(2), 239–244.

Chein, J. M., Moore, A. B., & Conway, A. R. (2011). Domain-general mechanisms of complex working memory span. *NeuroImage*, **54**(1), 550–559.

Conlin, J. A., Gathercole, S. E., & Adams, J. W. (2005). Children's working memory: Investigating performance limitations in complex span tasks. *Journal of Experimental Child Psychology*, **90**(4), 303–317.

Cowan, N. (2005). *Working memory capacity*. New York: Psychology Press.

Cowan, N. (2010). Multiple concurrent thoughts: The meaning and developmental neuropsychology of working memory. *Developmental Neuropsychology*, **35**(5), 447–474.

Crane, P. K., Narasimhalu, K., Gibbons, L. E., Pedraza, O., Mehta, K. M., Tang, Y., et al. (2008). Composite scores for executive function items: Demographic heterogeneity and relationships with quantitative magnetic resonance imaging. *Journal of the International Neuropsychological Society*, **14**(5), 746–759.

Delis, D. C., Kaplan, E., & Kramer, J. H. (2001). *Delis–Kaplan executive function system (DKEFS): Examiner's manual*. San Antonio, TX: The Psychological Corporation.

Dempster, F. N. (1981). Memory span: Sources of individual and developmental differences. *Psychological Bulletin*, **89**(1), 63–100.

Dennis, M., Spiegler, B. J., Hoffman, H. J., Hendrick, E. B., Humphreys, R. P., & Becker, L. E. (1991). Brain tumors in children and adolescents .1. Effects on working, associative and serial-order memory of IQ, Age at Tumor Onset and Age of Tumor. *Neuropsychologia*, **29**(9), 813–827.

D'Esposito, M., Postle, B. R., Ballard, D., & Lease, J. (1999). Maintenance versus manipulation of information held in working memory: An event-related fMRI study. *Brain and Cognition*, **41**(1), 66–86.

Dunn, L. M., & Dunn, D. M. (2007). *Peabody picture vocabulary test* (4th ed.). San Antonio, TX: Pearson.

Engle, R. W., Kane, M. J., & Tuholski, S. W. (1999). *Individual differences in working memory capacity and what they tell us about controlled attention, general fluid intelligence, and functions of the prefrontal cortex*. Cambridge: Cambridge University Press.

Fry, A. F., & Hale, S. (1996). Processing speed, working memory, and fluid intelligence: Evidence for a developmental cascade. *Psychological Science*, **7**(4), 237–241.

Fry, A. F., & Hale, S. (2000). Relationships among processing speed, working memory, and fluid intelligence in children. *Biological Psychology*, **54**(1–3), 1–34.

Garon, N., Bryson, S. E., & Smith, I. M. (2008). Executive function in preschoolers: A review using an integrative framework. *Psychological Bulletin*, **134**(1), 31–60.

Gathercole, S. E., Alloway, T. P., Willis, C., & Adams, A. M. (2006). Working memory in children with reading disabilities. *Journal of Experimental Child Psychology*, **93**(3), 265–281.

Gathercole, S. E., & Hitch, G. J. (1993). *Developmental changes in short-term memory: A revised working memory perspecitve*. Hove, England: Erlbaum.

Gathercole, S. E., Pickering, S. J., Ambridge, B., & Wearing, H. (2004). The structure of working memory from 4 to 15 years of age. *Developmental Psychology*, **40**(2), 177–190.

Geier, C. F., Garver, K., Terwilliger, R., & Luna, B. (2009). Development of working memory maintenance. *Journal of Neurophysiology*, **101**(1), 84–99.

Gold, J. M., Carpenter, C., Randolph, C., Goldberg, T. E., & Weinberger, D. R. (1997). Auditory working memory and Wisconsin Card Sorting Test performance in schizophrenia. *Archives of General Psychiatry*, **54**(2), 159–165.

Hitch, G. J., & Halliday, M. S. (1983). Working memory in children. *Philosophical Transactions of the Royal Society of London Series B: Biological Sciences*, **302**(1110), 325–340.

Holmes, J., Gathercole, S. E., & Dunning, D. L. (2009). Adaptive training leads to sustained enhancement of poor working memory in children. *Developmental Science*, **12**(4), F9–F15.

Kail, R., & Hall, L. K. (2001). Distinguishing short-term memory from working memory. *Memory & Cognition*, **29**(1), 1–9.

Kongs, S. K., Thompson, L. L., Iverson, G. L., & Heaton, R. K. (2000). *Wisconsin card sorting test-64 card version: Professional manual*. Odessa, FL: Psychological Assessment Resources.

Korkman, M., Kirk, U., & Kemp, S. (2007). *NEPSY* (2nd ed.). San Antonio, TX: Pearson.

Kwon, H., Reiss, A. L., & Menon, V. (2002). Neural basis of protracted developmental changes in visuo-spatial working memory. *Proceedings of the National Academy of Sciences of the United States of America*, **99**(20), 13336–13341.

Levin, H. S., Hanten, G., Zhang, L. F., Swank, P. R., Ewing-Cobbs, L., Dennis, M., et al. (2004). Changes in working memory after traumatic brain injury in children. *Neuropsychology*, **18**(2), 240–247.

McAuley, T., & White, D. A. (2011). A latent variables examination of processing speed, response inhibition, and working memory during typical development. *Journal of Experimental Child Psychology*, **108**(3), 453–468.

McNab, F., & Klingberg, T. (2008). Prefrontal cortex and basal ganglia control access to working memory. *Nature Neuroscience*, **11**(1), 103–107.

Miyake, A., Friedman, N. P., Emerson, M. J., Witzki, A. H., Howerter, A., & Wager, T. D. (2000). The unity and diversity of executive functions and their contributions to complex "frontal lobe" tasks: A latent variable analysis. *Cognitive Psychology*, **41**(1), 49–100.

Miyake, A., Friedman, N. P., Rettinger, D. A., Shah, P., & Hegarty, P. (2001). How are visuospatial working memory, executive functioning, and spatial abilities related? A latent-variable analysis. *Journal of Experimental Psychology: General*, **130**(4), 621–640.

Miyake, A., & Shah, P. (1999). *Models of working memory: Mechanisms of active maintenance and executive control*. New York: Cambridge University Press.

Munakata, Y. (2001). Graded representations in behavioral dissociations. *Trends in Cognitive Sciences*, **5**(7), 309–315.

Mungas, D., Reed, B. R., Tomaszewski Farias, S., & DeCarli, C. (2005). Criterion-referenced validity of a neuropsychological test battery: Equivalent performance in elderly Hispanics and non-Hispanic Whites. *Journal of the International Neuropsychological Society*, **11**(5), 620–630.

Mungas, D., Widaman, K., Zelazo, P. D., Tulsky, D. S., Heaton, R., Slotkin, J., et al. (This issue). Chapter 7—NIH Toolbox Cognitive Health Battery (CB): Factor Structure for 3- to 15-year-olds. *Monographs of the Society for Research in Child Development*.

Nelson, C. A., Monk, C. S., Lin, J., Carver, L. J., Thomas, K. M., & Truwit, C. L. (2000). Functional neuroanatomy of spatial working memory in children. *Developmental Psychology*, **36**(1), 109–116.

Nettelbeck, T., & Burns, N. R. (2010). Processing speed, working memory and reasoning ability from childhood to old age. *Personality and Individual Differences*, **48**(4), 379–384.

Nevo, E., & Breznitz, Z. (2011). Assessment of working memory components at 6 years of age as predictors of reading achievements a year later. *Journal of Experimental Child Psychology*, **109** (1), 73–90.

O'Hare, E. D., Lu, L. H., Houston, S. M., Bookheimer, S. Y., & Sowell, E. R. (2008). Neurodevelopmental changes in verbal working memory load-dependency: An fMRI investigation. *NeuroImage*, **42**(4), 1678–1685.

Osaka, N., Osaka, M., Kondo, H., Morishita, M., Fukuyama, H., & Shibasaki, H. (2004). The neural basis of executive function in working memory: An fMRI study based on individual differences. *NeuroImage*, **21**(2), 623–631.

Postle, B. R. (2006). Working memory as an emergent property of the mind and brain. *Neuroscience*, **139**(1), 23–38.

Reznick, J. S., Morrow, J. D., Goldman, B. D., & Snyder, J. (2004). The onset of working memory in infants. *Infancy*, **6**(1), 145–154.

Shing, Y. L., Lindenberger, U., Diamond, A., Li, S. C., & Davidson, M. C. (2010). Memory maintenance and inhibitory control differentiate from early childhood to adolescence. *Developmental Neuropsychology*, **35**(6), 679–697.

Smith-Spark, J. H., & Fisk, J. E. (2007). Working memory functioning in developmental dyslexia. *Memory*, **15**(1), 34–56.

St. Clair-Thompson, H. L. (2010). Backwards digit recall: A measure of short-term memory or working memory? *European Journal of Cognitive Psychology*, **22**, 286–296.

Thomason, M. E., Race, E., Burrows, B., Whitfield-Gabrieli, S., Glover, G. H., & Gabrieli, J. D. E. (2009). Development of spatial and verbal working memory capacity in the human brain. *Journal of Cognitive Neuroscience*, **21**(2), 316–332.

Thorell, L. B., Lindqvist, S., Bergman Nutley, S., Bohlin, G., & Klingberg, T. (2009). Training and transfer effects of executive functions in preschool children. *Developmental Science*, **12** (1), 106–113.

Towse, J. N., Hitch, G. J., & Hutton, U. (1998). A reevaluation of working memory capacity in children. *Journal of Memory and Language*, **39**(2), 195–217.

Tulsky, D. S., Saklofske, D. H., & Zhu, J. (2003). Revising a standard: An evaluation of the origin and development of the WAIS-III. In D. S. Tulsky, D. H. Saklofske, G. J. Chelune, R. K. Heaton, R. J. Ivnik, R. Bornstein, A. Prifitera, & M. F. Ledbetter (Eds.), *Clinical interpretation of the WAIS-III and WMS-III* (pp. 44–92). San Diego, CA: Academic Press.

Unsworth, N., & Engle, R. W. (2007). The nature of individual differences in working memory capacity: Active maintenance in primary memory and controlled search from secondary memory. *Psychological Review*, **114**(1), 104–132.

Vicari, S., Caravale, B., Carlesimo, G. A., Casadei, A. M., & Allemand, F. (2004). Spatial working memory deficits in children at ages 3–4 who were low birth weight, preterm infants. *Neuropsychology*, **18**(4), 673–678.

Wager, T. D., & Smith, E. E. (2003). Neuroimaging studies of working memory: A meta-analysis. *Cognitive Affective and Behavioral Neuroscience*, **3**(4), 255–274.

Wechsler, D. (1997). *Wechsler Adult Intelligence Scale III*. San Antonio, TX: Harcourt Assessment.

Wechsler, D. (2003). *WISC-IV administration and scoring manual*. San Antonio, TX: PsychCorp.

Wechsler, D. (2008). *Wechsler Adult Intelligence Scale IV*. San Antonio, TX: Harcourt Assessment.

Weintraub, S., Bauer, P. J., Zelazo, P. D., Wallner-Allen, K., Dikmen, S., Heaton, R. K., et al. (This issue). Chapter 1—NIH Toolbox Cognition Battery (CB): Introduction and Pediatric Data. *Monographs of the Society for Research in Child Development*.

Wiebe, S. A., Espy, K. A., & Charak, D. (2008). Using confirmatory factor analysis to understand executive control in preschool children: I. Latent structure. *Developmental Psychology*, **44**(2), 575–587.

Wiebe, S. A., Sheffield, T., Nelson, J. M., Clark, C. A., Chevalier, N., & Espy, K. A. (2011). The structure of executive function in 3-year-olds. *Journal of Experimental Child Psychology*, **108**(3), 436–452.

Willcutt, E. G., Doyle, A. E., Nigg, J. T., Faraone, S. V., & Pennington, B. F. (2005). Validity of the executive function theory of attention-deficit/hyperactivity disorder: A meta-analytic review. *Biological Psychiatry*, **57**(11), 1336–1346.

Williams, D. L., Goldstein, G., & Minshew, N. J. (2006). The profile of memory function in children with autism. *Neuropsychology*, **20**(1), 21–29.

VI. NIH TOOLBOX COGNITION BATTERY (CB): MEASURING PROCESSING SPEED

Noelle E. Carlozzi, David S. Tulsky, Robert V. Kail, and Jennifer L. Beaumont

ABSTRACT This chapter focuses on the Toolbox Pattern Comparison Processing Speed Test, which was developed to assess processing speed within the NIH Toolbox Cognition Battery (CB). We describe the development of the test, highlighting its utility in children. In addition, we examine descriptive data, test–retest reliability, validity, and preliminary work creating a composite index of processing speed. Results indicated that most children were able to understand the basic concepts of the Toolbox Pattern Comparison Processing Speed Test. Further, test–retest reliability was excellent. Analyses examining convergent and discriminant validity provided support for the utility of the test as a measure of processing speed. Finally, analyses comparing and combining scores on the Toolbox Pattern Comparison Processing Speed Test with other measures of simple reaction time from the NIH Toolbox CB indicated that a Processing Speed Composite score performed better than any test examined in isolation. Taken together, the Toolbox Pattern Comparison Processing Speed Test appears to exhibit a number of strengths: it is child-friendly and engaging, short and easy to administer, and has good construct validity, especially when used as part of a composite score.

In this chapter, we discuss the Toolbox Pattern Comparison Processing Speed Test, the measure designed to assess processing speed.

Subdomain Definition

Processing speed is an extremely important developmental construct. Age differences in speeded responses are robust and reliable across the lifespan. On simple tasks, reaction time (RT) generally decreases systematically from infancy through childhood and adolescence, reaching a minimum

---

Corresponding author: Noelle E. Carlozzi, Department of Physical Medicine and Rehabilitation, Center for Rehabilitation Outcomes and Assessment Research, North Campus Research Complex, Building 520, 2800 Plymouth Road, Ann Arbor, MI 48109-2800, email: carlozzi@med.umich.edu

in young adulthood; thereafter, RT increases modestly during middle age, and more substantially in old age. The developmental profile of increasing RT speed between birth and young adulthood can be exemplified by three different types of studies. First, on a simple RT task in which children respond to an auditory or visual stimulus by pressing a key, RTs are much greater for children than for adolescents, whose RTs are somewhat larger than those for adults (Kail, 1991). Second, judging whether pairs of pictures are identical in name takes longer than judging whether they are identical in appearance (Kail, 1991); discrepancies in RT between these two types of tasks times are smallest for young adults, somewhat larger for adolescents, and much larger for children (Kail, 1991). Finally, saccadic eye movements to targets in peripheral vision become faster with age, substantially so in the first year of life and more gradually thereafter (Canfield, Smith, Brezsnyak, & Snow, 1997; Luna, Garver, Urban, Lazar, & Sweeney, 2004).

Importance During Childhood

The developmental profile of RT is not restricted to motor processing. Instead, reductions in RT are evident in a broad range of cognitive processes, including executive function (see Zelazo et al., Chapter 2, this volume) and episodic memory (see Bauer et al., Chapter 3, this volume). Consequently, changes in RT are often described as developmental changes in information processing speed (Kail, 2008; Kail & Salthouse, 1994). Evidence shows that increases in processing speed are associated with age-related improvements in performance on a variety of cognitive tasks, including reading, memory, arithmetic problem solving, way-finding, and reasoning (Kail, 2004, 2008). In some cases, processing speed accounts statistically for all of the variance in age-related cognitive changes (i.e., significant associations between age and cognitive skill disappear when processing speed is partialled out). In addition, longitudinal research shows that measures of processing speed administered during infancy predict mental development in the preschool years (Rose, Feldman, Jankowski, & Van Rossem, 2008).

Cognitive Processing and Biological Substrates

When measuring processing speed across the lifespan, it is important to consider the cognitive processes that drive increases in processing speed, as well as their biological substrates. First, the fact that speeds of a number of different processes increase with age does not necessarily implicate a common mechanism. One possibility—building on the well-established link between repeated practice and RT (Newell & Rosenbloom, 1981) and the view of young children as universal novices (Brown & DeLoache, 1978)—is that speeds of individual processes develop at distinct rates, each reflecting task-relevant experience. Following this logic, the usual correlation between age and processing speed is seen as a byproduct of correlations between age/experience and experience/speed. Another possibility is that developmental increases in processing speed reflect some underlying systemic change (i.e., change in a fundamental property of the developing cognitive architecture). In fact, processing speeds in different domains increase at a common rate (Kail, 1986, 1988, 1991), supporting the notion of a global mechanism. In addition, factor-analytic studies provide evidence that processing speed measures are significantly intercorrelated and can be distinguished from other related cognitive constructs such as response inhibition, working memory, and cognitive control throughout childhood and adolescence (Demetriou, Mouyi, & Spanoudis, 2008; McAuley & White, 2011).

While a number of cognitive processes influence processing speed, it is also important to consider the biological substrates of this behavior. Specifically, there is indirect evidence that increases in processing speed may be a byproduct of neural changes. For example, children with neural impairments including developmental disability (Nettelbeck & Wilson, 1997), closed head injury (Brookshire, Levin, Song, & Zhang, 2004), and phenylketonuria (Anderson et al., 2007) have slower processing speed relative to their typically developing age-mates. In addition, long-term survivors of childhood acute lymphoblastic leukemia that have been treated with radiation (resulting in myelin damage) have slower processing speed than controls (Schatz, Kramer, Ablin, & Matthay, 2000, 2004). There also is evidence from neuroimaging studies that greater white matter (used as an index of myelination) is associated with faster processing (Soria-Pastor et al., 2008), but only for subgroups of participants (Silveri, Tzilos, & Yurgelun-Todd, 2008) or subsets of speeded tasks (Mabbott, Noseworthy, Bouffet, Laughlin, & Rockel, 2006). Taken together, results are consistent with the claim that neural development contributes to increases in processing speed, but more research is needed to identify the specific neural elements that are involved.

Measuring Processing Speed

Two approaches have been used to measure processing speed in children, adolescents, and adults. One uses tasks from experimental psychology in which a stimulus is presented and participants respond by selecting one of two alternatives, typically by pressing a button or a key on a keyboard. Tasks are constructed to include different within-participant conditions to isolate speeds of specific processes. The simplest version of this task would include two conditions. In one, participants respond whenever any stimulus appears. In the other, they make one response for certain stimuli (e.g., upper-case letters) but another response for other stimuli (e.g., lower-case letters). Responses are slower in the second condition and the difference is said to reflect the additional time for participants to make a decision, such as, whether the letter was upper or lower case. Tasks built on this logic are commonplace when investigators wish to focus on particular processes. However, these tasks are time-consuming because many trials are needed within each condition to estimate RTs accurately. Even then, the data rarely achieve accepted psychometric levels of reliability. In addition, children are often bored by the repetitive nature of these tasks, which can cause their performance to deteriorate over the duration of the task.

Consequently, many investigators rely upon psychometric measures of perceptual speed. A typical test of this sort is the Cross Out task from the Woodcock–Johnson Tests of Cognitive Ability. In this test, there are 30 rows with a target geometric figure at the left end of a row and 19 similar figures to the right. For example, one row consists of a triangle enclosing a single dot and the 19 figures to the right depict triangles with various objects (e.g., a single dot, three dots) in the interior. The participant places a line through the five figures of the 19 that are identical to the target figure at the left. The performance measure is the number of rows accurately completed in 3 min. Performance on these and similar tasks is highly reliable (e.g., test–retest reliabilities for the Cross Out tasks are .64–.73, for children and adolescents).

Toolbox Measurement: Development of the Toolbox Pattern Comparison Processing Speed Test

The Toolbox Pattern Comparison Processing Speed Test is modeled directly on Salthouse's Pattern Comparison Task (Salthouse, Babcock, & Shaw, 1991), an extensively researched assessment of choice RT in older adults but also is similar to both experimental and psychometric measures (described previously) that have been used to measure processing speed in children. In the Toolbox Pattern Comparison Processing Speed Test, participants are asked to identify whether two visual patterns are the "same" or "not the same." Scores reflect the number of correct responses within a finite time frame.

For an initial pilot study, eight 3-year-old children were recruited from a local nursery school to examine task feasibility. Items were administered on the computer, and examiners recorded verbal responses on a separate record form. Patterns were either identical or varied on one of three dimensions: adding/taking something away, one versus many, or changing positions. Scores reflected the number of correct items (of a possible 251) completed in 3 min.

Three-year-olds received average scores of 44.4 ($SD = 12.3$; range 25–59). In addition, participants made an average of 9.5 errors ($SD = 12.3$; range 3–13). When errors were tallied, there were 8 items that were potentially problematic (where four or more participants made errors). From these data, the task was revised to allow children to indicate responses via touchscreen, minimizing the bias introduced by an examiner needing to both record responses and prompt the next item once a response was provided. In addition, we decided to eliminate discriminations that involved changing positions, as there were not very many items along this dimension.

In a second ("prevalidation") pilot study, children were asked to identify whether two visual patterns are the "same" or "not the same": children ages 3–7 years indicated responses by pressing either a "smiley face button" or "frown face button" on the touchscreen; children ages 8–14 years indicated responses using a "yes" or "no" button on the touchscreen. Patterns were either identical or varied on one of three dimensions: color, adding/taking something away, or one versus many. We examined participants ages 3–4 years ($n = 35$), 5–7 years ($n = 26$), and 8–14 years ($n = 28$). In addition, we utilized three different time cut-offs (60, 90, or 120 sec) to determine optimal test administration time. Test–retest reliability was in the adequate range ($ICC = .56-.69$); performance was generally comparable regardless of the test administration time. We decided to move ahead using the 90 sec version of the test. In addition, items with less than 75% correct response rates were dropped, and findings provided support for deleting the one versus many discrimination for children ages 3–7 years. The 90 sec version of the test was administered in a validation study that included the full age range of the NIH Toolbox, ages 3–85 years. This monograph focuses on the results of this study for children and young adolescents ages 3–15 years. The validation data from the adult and elderly populations will be published in a separate series of papers so that each population can be addressed in greater depth.

METHOD

Participants

The participants in the validation study are described in detail in Weintraub et al. (Chapter 1, this volume; Table 3). Eighteen children did not complete the task; all were ages 3–5 years. Reasons included lack of attention or alertness or general noncompliance. One 15-year-old had an outlying score of zero and was excluded from analysis.

Toolbox Measures

Participants were tested with the Toolbox Pattern Comparison Processing Speed Test. In addition, RT scores from other NIHTB-CB measures (Toolbox

Dimensional Change Card Sort [DCCS] Test and the Toolbox Flanker Inhibitory Control and Attention Test) were utilized to generate a Processing Speed Composite score.

The Toolbox Pattern Comparison Processing Speed Test

The Toolbox Pattern Comparison Processing Speed Test provides a measure of processing speed. The validation version of this measure required participants to identify whether two visual patterns are the "same" or "not the same." Children registered their responses as described above for the second, "prevalidation" pilot study. Patterns were either identical or varied on one of three dimensions: color (all ages), adding/taking something away (all ages), or one versus many (only ages 8–15 years; see Figure 11). Scores reflected the number of correct items (of a possible 104 for ages 3–7 years and 130 for ages 8–15 years) completed in 90 sec; items were designed to minimize the number of errors that were made (i.e., items with less than 75% accuracy during pilot testing and prevalidation were not included in the final version of this task).

Processing Speed Composite

The processing speed composite was composed of the Toolbox Pattern Comparison Processing Speed Test and two other CB measures, the Toolbox Dimensional Change Card Sort (DCCS) and the Toolbox Flanker Inhibitory Control and Attention Test, both of which are described in detail in Zelazo et al. (Chapter 2, this volume). For the composite measure, we examined mean RT for all DCCS (frequent and nonfrequent) and all Flanker (congruent and incongruent) trials.

Validation Measures

In addition to the CB measures, we administered several other tasks to test convergent (Wechsler Preschool and Primary Scale of Intelligence, 3rd Edition or Wechsler Intelligence Scale for Children, 4th Edition Processing Speed Composite, Paced Auditory Serial Addition Test) and discriminant

Color Discrimination   Adding/Taking Something Away   One versus Many

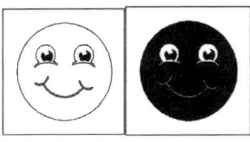 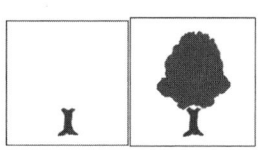 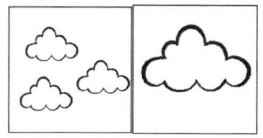

FIGURE 11.—Examples of varied dimensions for discriminations on the Toolbox Pattern Comparison Processing Speed Test.
Note. Discriminations are made for color (ages 3–15 years), adding something versus taking something away (ages 3–15 years), and one versus many (ages 8–15 years).

validity (Wechsler Intelligence Scale for Children, 4th Edition Letter-Number Sequencing, Peabody Picture Vocabulary Test, 4th Edition, PPVT-IV).

Convergent Validity

Participants ages 5–6 years completed the Wechsler Preschool and Primary Scale of Intelligence, 3rd Edition (WPPSI-III) and participants ages 8–15 years completed the Wechsler Intelligence Scale for Children, 4th Edition (WISC-IV) Processing Speed Composite tasks (Wechsler, 2002, 2004). The Processing Speed Composite is a composite score that combines performance on WPPSI-III/WISC-IV Coding and WPPSI-III/WISC-IV Symbol Search. WPPSI-III/WISC-IV Coding requires the participant to associate numbers and symbols using a key. Scores reflect number of items completed correctly in 120 sec (maximum 135). WPPSI-III/WISC-IV Symbol Search requires the participant to identify whether target symbols (two symbols) are part of a group of five symbols. Scores reflect number correct minus number incorrect in 120 sec (maximum 60). This composite score averages performance on WPPSI-III/WISC-IV Coding and WPPSI-III/WISC-IV Symbol Search; it does not adjust for age (as does the WPPSI-III/WISC-IV Processing Speed Index).

Participants ages 8–15 years completed the Paced Auditory Serial Addition Test (PASAT; Gronwall, 1977). The PASAT is a measure of cognitive function that specifically assesses auditory information processing speed, sustained attention, and calculation ability. Single digits are presented every 2 sec and the participant must add each new digit to the one immediately prior to it. The test result is the number of correct sums given (maximum 50).

Discriminant Validity

Participants ages 3–15 years completed the PPVT-IV (Dunn & Dunn, 2007). The PPVT-IV provides a measure of receptive vocabulary and word retrieval. Participants are asked to identify which of four pictures is denoted by a specific word. Scores are based on the number correct (maximum 228).

Participants ages 8–15 years completed the WISC-IV Letter-Number Sequencing test (Wechsler, 2008). In this test, participants are presented with a mixed list of numbers and letters, and their task is first to repeat the list by saying the numbers in ascending order and then to repeat the letters in alphabetical order; it provides a measure of working memory. Scores reflect the number of correct responses (maximum 30 points), with higher scores indicating better performance.

Data Analysis

For all tests, scaled scores were created by first ranking the raw scores, next applying a normative transformation to the ranks to create a standard normal distribution, and finally rescaling the distribution to have a mean of 10 and a standard deviation of 3. The WPPSI-III/WISC-IV Processing Speed Composite described above was calculated by averaging the individual scaled scores and then renormalizing.

We examined the relations between the Toolbox Pattern Comparison Processing Speed Test and age, test–retest reliability, and construct validity. Pearson correlation coefficients were used to assess the relation between age and Toolbox Pattern Comparison Processing Speed Test performance. Intraclass correlation coefficients (*ICC*) were calculated to evaluate test–retest reliability. Convergent validity was assessed via Pearson correlation coefficients between the Toolbox Pattern Comparison Processing Speed Test and established measures of the same construct (i.e., WPPSI-III/WISC-IV Composite Score and PASAT). Evidence of discriminant validity consisted of lower correlations with selected validation measures of *different* cognitive constructs: working memory (WISC-IV Letter Number Sequencing) and receptive vocabulary (PPVT-IV).

We also conducted analyses to create a composite score of processing speed using multiple measures from the CB. For these analyses, we compared different summary scores that reflected processing speed estimates using (1) the Toolbox Pattern Comparison Processing Speed Test, (2) the Toolbox DCCS (mean RT on all trials, including frequent and infrequent), (3) the Toolbox Flanker Inhibitory Control and Attention Test (mean RT on all trials, including congruent and incongruent), as well as (4) the average of these three scores. Specifically, we examined the relations of this composite score with our validation measures (WPPSI-III/WISC-IV Processing Speed Composite and the PASAT). In addition, we examined test–retest reliability for our composite score.

RESULTS

Age Effects

Figure 12 provides a graphic presentation of performance on the Toolbox Pattern Comparison Processing Speed Test from ages 3 to 15 years. A positive association between age and the Toolbox Pattern Comparison Processing Speed Test ($r(187) = .77; p < .0001$) was seen in children, and a quadratic model provided the best fit of the data, with $R^2 = .66$. Pairwise comparisons between age groups are reported in Appendix A.

Test–Retest Reliability

Overall *ICC* for the Toolbox Pattern Comparison Processing Speed Test (ages 3–15 years) was .84 (95% CI: .75, .90; $p < .0001$).

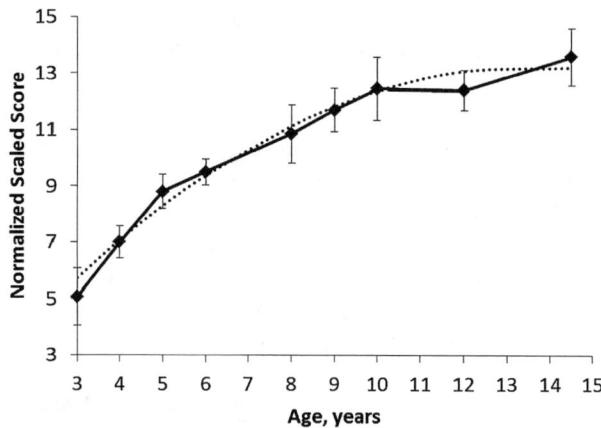

FIGURE 12.—Normalized scaled scores on the Toolbox Pattern Comparison Processing Speed Test across age groups. Error bars are ±2 standard errors. Best-fitting polynomial curve is also shown (see text).

Effect of Repeated Testing

Practice effects were computed as the difference between test and retest normalized scaled scores, with significance of the effect being tested with t tests for dependent means. For the total child group (ages 3–15 years, $n = 66$), the Toolbox Pattern Comparison Processing Speed Test showed a practice effect over an average 2-week test–retest interval: *mean practice effect* $= .67$, $SD = 1.60$, $t(58) = 3.22$, $p = .002$.

Convergent and Discriminant Validity

Table 11 shows results for convergent and discriminant validity for ages 3–15 years; please note that we did not administer measures of processing speed for children under the age of 5. Correlations for convergent validity ranged from $r = .31$ to $r = .43$ (all $p \leq .01$), suggesting that the Toolbox Pattern Comparison Processing Speed Test has adequate convergent validity and is indeed tapping processing speed. Correlations with discriminant validity measures of working memory and receptive vocabulary ranged from $r = .20$ to $r = .44$. Discriminant correlations did not differ significantly from the corresponding convergent correlations.

Processing Speed Composite Score

Three measures of processing speed (Toolbox Pattern Comparison Processing Speed Test, and mean RT from all DCCS and Flanker trials) were

TABLE 11

Pearson Correlations Between the Toolbox Pattern Comparison Processing Speed Test and Convergent and Discriminant Validation Measures

Validation Measure	Toolbox Pattern Comparison Processing Speed Test					
	(Ages 3–6 years)			(Ages 8–15 years)		
	df	r	p-Value	df	r	p-Value
Convergent Validity Measures						
WPPSI-III/WISC-IV Processing Speed Composite[a]	55	.43	<.0001	83	.40	<.0001
PASAT	—	—	—	82	.39	<.0001
Discriminant Validity Measures						
PPVT-IV	97	.44	<.0001	84	.36	<.0001
WAIS-IV Letter-Number Sequencing	—	—	—	82	.20	.07

Note. Unadjusted scaled scores were utilized in analyses. WPPSI-III, Wechsler Preschool and Primary Scale of Intelligence, 3rd Edition; WISC-IV, Wechsler Intelligence Scale for Children, 4th Edition; PASAT, Paced Auditory Serial Attention Test; PPVT-IV, Peabody Picture Vocabulary Test-4th Edition; WAIS-IV, Wechsler Adult Scale of Intelligence, 4th Edition.
[a]WISC-IV Processing Speed Composite was calculated for children ages 5–6 years.
© 2006–2012 National Institutes of Health and Northwestern University.

utilized to create an NIH Toolbox Processing Speed Composite Score. The individual scores (Toolbox Pattern Comparison Processing Speed, Toolbox DCCS, and Toolbox Flanker Inhibitory Control and Attention Test mean RT) and the Processing Speed Composite Score demonstrated similar correlations with age ($r = .77–.83$; see Table 12) and test–retest reliabilities ($r = .84–.87$; see Table 12). The NIH Toolbox Processing Speed Composite demonstrated higher correlations with established measures than did the Toolbox Pattern Comparison Processing Speed Test (see Table 13).

DISCUSSION

In this chapter we described the development of the Toolbox Pattern Comparison Processing Speed Test from the NIH Toolbox Cognition Battery and explored its utility in children as well as its use as a measure of processing speed. Data were presented for 208 children (age 3–15 years) on three important psychometric characteristics: sensitivity to cognitive improvement during childhood, test–retest reliability, and construct validity tested against established measures in the field. In addition, data were presented that

TABLE 12

Pearson Age-Related Correlations and Test–Retest Correlations (Intraclass Correlations; ICC) for the NIH Toolbox Pattern Comparison Processing Speed Test and the NIH Toolbox Processing Speed Composite Score (Using Toolbox Pattern Comparison Processing Speed Test, Toolbox DCCS, and Toolbox Flanker) for Children Ages 3 to 15 Years

NIH Toolbox Cognition Domain/Instrument	Age-related correlations		Test–retest correlations	
	df	r	df	ICC
Toolbox Pattern Comparison Processing Speed Test	187	.77	57	.84
NIH Toolbox Processing Speed Composite	203	.83	64	.88

Note. © 2006–2012 National Institutes of Health and Northwestern University. All $ps < .0001$.

explore the optimal method of estimating processing speed within the NIH Toolbox using both the Toolbox Pattern Comparison Processing Speed Test, as well as two other cognitive measures from the NIH Toolbox that include simple RT assessment (DCCS and Flanker). As noted above, results indicated that most children were able to understand the basic concepts of the Toolbox Pattern Comparison Processing Speed Test. Further, test–retest reliability was excellent.

In addition, evidence for test validity was supported by multiple findings. Specifically, as mentioned earlier, processing speed follows a well-defined developmental trajectory: it increases systematically through childhood and adolescence, peaks in young adulthood, slows modestly during middle age, and more substantially in older age (Kail, 1991, 2008; Kail & Salthouse, 1994). Findings from this study demonstrate similar age-related performance patterns across childhood.

Analyses examining the convergent and discriminant validity of the Toolbox Pattern Comparison Processing Speed Test also provided some support for the utility of this task as a measure of processing speed. Specifically, the new test demonstrated moderate relations with other measures that examine processing speed (i.e., a composite score based on WPPSI-III/WISC-IV Coding and Symbol Search, and the PASAT), and slightly less strong associations with measures that assess other domains of cognitive function (working memory as assessed by WISC-IV Letter-Number Sequencing and language as assessed by the PPVT-IV). The moderate relations with convergent validity measures were lower than we had anticipated, which may be attributed to the fact that responses were recorded via touchscreen. The touchscreen introduced some unanticipated response variability—even though all participants were instructed to respond "as quickly as possible,"

TABLE 13
PEARSON CORRELATIONS BETWEEN NIH TOOLBOX PROCESSING SPEED COMPOSITE SCORE (USING TOOLBOX PATTERN COMPARISON PROCESSING SPEED TEST, TOOLBOX DCCS, AND TOOLBOX FLANKER) AND VALIDATION MEASURES

	Validation Measure											
	WPPSI-III/WISC-IV Processing Speed Composite						PASAT			PPVT-IV		
	(Ages 5–6)			(Ages 8–15)			(Ages 8–15)			(Ages 3–15)		
Processing Speed Estimate	r	df	p-Value	r	df	p-Value	r	df	p-Value	r	df	p-Value
Toolbox Pattern Comparison Processing Speed Test	.40	55	<.002	.39	83	<.0001	.39	82	<.0002	.73	183	<.0001
NIH Toolbox Processing Speed Composite	.37	56	<.004	.44	84	<.0001	.34	83	<.001	.82	198	<.0001

Note. WPPSI-III, Wechsler Preschool and Primary Scale of Intelligence, 3rd Edition; WISC-IV, Wechsler Intelligence Scale for Children, 4th Edition; PASAT, Paced Auditory Serial Attention Test; PPVT-IV, Peabody Picture Vocabulary Test-4th Edition.

some individuals hovered over the response buttons, whereas others returned a resting position (by lowering their hand or placing it on the table in between trials). As a result of these findings we have made additional changes to this measure that will require individuals to respond using a computer keyboard. These changes will be implemented for the norming study. Assuming that results from the norming study are promising, additional validation data will be needed to better establish convergent validity.

Finally, when three indices of processing speed were combined (Toolbox Pattern Comparison Processing Speed scores, Toolbox DCCS RT, and Toolbox Flanker Inhibitory Control and Attention Test RT), relations between the NIH Toolbox Processing Speed Composite and the validation measures were higher than those between the Toolbox Pattern Comparison Processing Speed Test (alone) and the validation measures. We anticipate that the NIH Toolbox Processing Speed composite score will be refined during the norming phase of the NIH Toolbox study. It is likely that this score will be more robust, more sensitive, and include less measurement error, than any processing speed score derived from a single test. Ultimately, this type of composite score should have utility in clinical trials and longitudinal research involving participants across a broad age range.[3]

REFERENCES

Anderson, P. J., Wood, S. J., Francis, D. E., Coleman, L., Anderson, V., & Boneh, A. (2007). Are neuropsychological impairments in children with early-treated phenylketonuria (PKU) related to white matter abnormalities or elevated phenylalanine levels? *Developmental Neuropsychology*, **32**(2), 645–668.

Bauer, P. J., Dikmen, S., Heaton, R., Mungas, D., Slotkin, J., & Beaumont, J. L. (This issue). Chapter 3—NIH Toolbox Cognition Battery (CHB): Measuring episodic memory. *Monographs of the Society for Research in Child Development*.

Brookshire, B., Levin, H. S., Song, J., & Zhang, L. (2004). Components of executive function in typically developing and head-injured children. *Developmental Neuropsychology*, **25**(1–2), 61–83.

Brown, A., & DeLoache, J. S. (1978). Skills, plans and self-regulation. In R. Siegler (Ed.), *Children's thinking: What develops?* (pp. 3–35). Hillsdale, NJ: Erlbaum.

Canfield, R. L., Smith, E. G., Brezsnyak, M. P., & Snow, K. L. (1997). Information processing through the first year of life: A longitudinal study using the visual expectation paradigm. *Monographs of the Society for Research in Child Development*, **62**(2), 1–145.

Demetriou, A., Mouyi, A., & Spanoudis, G. (2008). Modelling the structure and development of g. *Intelligence*, **36**(5), 437–454.

Dunn, L. M., & Dunn, D. M. (2007). *Peabody Picture Vocabulary Test* (4th ed.). San Antonio, TX: Pearson.

Gronwall, D. M. A. (1977). Paced Auditory Serial-Addition Task—Measure of Recovery from Concussion. *Perceptual and Motor Skills*, **44**(2), 367–373.

Kail, R. V. (1986). Sources of age differences in speed of processing. *Child Development*, **57**(4), 969–987.

Kail, R. V. (1988). Developmental functions for speeds of cognitive processes. *Journal of Experimental Child Psychology*, **45**(3), 339–364.

Kail, R. V. (1991). Processing time declines exponentially during childhood and adolescence. *Developmental Psychology*, **27**(2), 259–266.

Kail, R. V. (2004). Cognitive development includes global and domain-specific processes. *Merrill-Palmer Quarterly*, **50**(4), 445–455.

Kail, R. V. (2008). *Speed of processing in childhood and adolescence: Nature, consequences, and implications for understanding atypical development.* New York: Taylor and Francis.

Kail, R. V., & Miller, C. A. (2006). Developmental change in processing speed: Domain specificity and stability during childhood and adolescence. *Journal of Cognition and Development*, **7**, 119–137.

Kail, R. V., & Salthouse, T. A. (1994). Processing speed as a mental-capacity. *Acta Psychologica*, **86**(2–3), 199–225.

Kiselev, S., Espy, K. A., & Sheffield, T. (2009). Age-related differences in reaction time task performance in young children. *Journal of Experimental Child Psychology*, **102**, 150–166.

Luna, B., Garver, K. E., Urban, T. A., Lazar, N. A., & Sweeney, J. A. (2004). Maturation of cognitive processes from late childhood to adulthood. *Child Development*, **75**(5), 1357–1372.

Mabbott, D. J., Noseworthy, M., Bouffet, E., Laughlin, S., & Rockel, C. (2006). White matter growth as a mechanism of cognitive development in children. *NeuroImage*, **33**(3), 936–946.

McAuley, T., & White, D. A. (2011). A latent variables examination of processing speed, response inhibition, and working memory during typical development. *Journal of Experimental Child Psychology*, **108**(3), 453–468.

Nettelbeck, T., & Wilson, C. (1997). Speed of information processing and cognition. In W. E. MacLean Jr (Ed.), *Ellis' handbook of mental deficiency, psychological theory and research* (3rd ed., pp. 245–274). Mahwah, NJ: Erlbaum.

Newell, A., & Rosenbloom, P. S. (1981). *Mechanisms of skill acquisition and the law of practice.* Hillsdale, NJ: Erlbaum.

Rose, S. A., Feldman, J. F., Jankowski, J. J., & Van Rossem, R. (2008). A cognitive cascade in infancy: Pathways from prematurity to later mental development. *Intelligence*, **36**(4), 367–378.

Roth, C. (1983). Factors affecting developmental changes in the speed of processing. *Journal of Experimental Child Psychology*, **35**, 509–528.

Salthouse, T. A., Babcock, R. L., & Shaw, R. J. (1991). Effects of adult age on structural and operational capacities in working memory. *Psychology and Aging*, **6**(1), 118–127.

Schatz, J., Kramer, J. H., Ablin, A., & Matthay, K. K. (2000). Processing speed, working memory, and IQ: A developmental model of cognitive deficits following cranial radiation therapy. *Neuropsychology*, **14**(2), 189–200.

Schatz, J., Kramer, J. H., Ablin, A. R., & Matthay, K. K. (2004). Visual attention in long-term survivors of leukemia receiving cranial radiation therapy. *Journal of the International Neuropsychological Society*, **10**(2), 211–220.

Silveri, M. M., Tzilos, G. K., & Yurgelun-Todd, D. A. (2008). Relationship between white matter volume and cognitive performance during adolescence: Effects of age, sex and risk for drug use. *Addiction*, **103**(9), 1509–1520.

Soria-Pastor, S., Gimenez, M., Narberhaus, A., Falcon, C., Botet, F., Bargallo, N., et al. (2008). Patterns of cerebral white matter damage and cognitive impairment in adolescents born very preterm. *International Journal of Developmental Neuroscience,* **26**(7), 647–654.

Wechsler, D. (2002). *The Wechsler Preschool and Primary Scale of Intelligence* (3rd ed.). San Antonio, TX: The Psychological Corporation.

Wechsler, D. (2004). *The Wechsler Intelligence Scale for Children* (4th ed.). San Antonio, TX: The Psychological Corporation.

Wechsler, D. (2008). *Wechsler Adult Intelligence Scale IV.* San Antonio, TX: Harcourt Assessment.

Weintraub, S., Bauer, P. J., Zelazo, P. D., Wallner-Allen, K., Dikmen, S., Heaton, R. K., et al. (This issue). Chapter 1—NIH Toolbox Cognition Battery (CB): Introduction and pediatric data. *Monographs of the Society for Research in Child Development.*

Zelazo, P. D., Anderson, J. E., Richler, J., Wallner-Allen, K., Beaumont, J. L., & Weintraub, S. (This issue). Chapter 2—NIH Toolbox Cognition Battery (CB): Measuring executive function and attention. *Monographs of the Society for Research in Child Development.*

NOTE

3. Findings of this sort do not undermine claims that task-specific experiences contribute to age-related change in processing speed. Indeed, there is evidence that speeds of some processes develop at different rates from the global mechanism (Kail & Miller, 2006; Kiselev, Espy, & Sheffield, 2009) and that expertise can enhance children's processing speed (Roth, 1983). It is plausible that speeds of many processes develop at a common rate reflecting the same underlying mechanism but that speeds of other processes develop at different rates, reflecting distinct mechanisms.

VII. NIH TOOLBOX COGNITION BATTERY (CB): FACTOR STRUCTURE FOR 3 TO 15 YEAR OLDS

Dan Mungas, Keith Widaman, Philip David Zelazo, David Tulsky, Robert K. Heaton, Jerry Slotkin, David L. Blitz, and Richard C. Gershon

ABSTRACT Confirmatory factor analysis was used the evaluate the dimensional structure underlying the NIH Toolbox Cognition Battery (CB) and the measures chosen to serve as concurrent validity criteria for the NIH Toolbox CB. These results were used to evaluate the convergent and discriminant validity of the CB in children ranging from 3 to 15 years of age. Results were evaluated separately for a 3- to 6-year-old group and a 8- to 15-year-old group because different validation measures were used in these age groups. Three distinct dimensions were found for the 3- to 6-year-old group: Vocabulary, Reading, and Fluid Abilities. Five dimensions were found for 8–15 year olds: Vocabulary, Reading, Episodic Memory, Working Memory, and Executive Function/Processing Speed. CB measures and their validation analogues consistently defined common factors in a pattern that broadly supported the convergent and discriminant validity of the CB, but results showed higher intercorrelation and less differentiation of cognitive dimensions in younger than in older children and in older children compared with adults. Age was strongly related to the cognitive dimensions underlying test performance in both groups of children and results are consistent with broader literature showing increasing differentiation of cognitive abilities associated with the rapid brain development that occurs from early childhood into adulthood.

In this chapter, we discuss convergent and discriminant validity of the NIH Toolbox Cognition Battery (CB). This is accomplished using confirmatory factor analysis (CFA) to identify the dimensions underlying the CB tests and established validation measures, and to test the hypothesis

---

Corresponding author: Dan Mungas, Department of Neurology, 4860 Y Street, Suite 3700, Sacramento, CA 95817, email: dmmungas@ucdavis.edu

that the CB tests measure the specific domains they were designed to measure.

Cognition undergoes rapid developmental changes across the 3- to 15-year age range related to brain development and extensive environmental input, especially formal education, which is designed to develop cognitive skills and expand knowledge. An overarching goal of the CB is to be able to assess cognitive abilities across the life span, and this presupposes that the same abilities are being measured in the same way at different ages. Consequently, a critical part of the construct validation tests whether expected relations with widely used instruments are present at different ages.

Reasons to Expect Age-Related Differences in Factor Structure

Construct validity begins with a conceptual model that describes the expected relations between domains being measured and specific tests used to measure those domains. The CB was designed to assess six specific subdomains: executive function (with tests of cognitive flexibility, inhibitory control, and attention), episodic memory, language (vocabulary), reading, working memory, and processing speed. This test development model provides a conceptual foundation for the construct validation of the CB. However, developmental changes in the structure of cognition that occur across childhood have implications for specific hypotheses deriving from this conceptual model.

A great deal of brain development occurs before birth, but it is now clear that brain development is a protracted process, with major changes taking place during the preschool years and continuing into adolescence and early adulthood. Indeed, recent technological advances have allowed unprecedented opportunities to observe detailed developmental changes in the living brain, and researchers are beginning to chart the way in which developmental changes (both progressive and regressive) in specific neural systems are related to changes in different aspects of cognitive function.

Considerable research supports the suggestion that key aspects of neurocognitive development involve the experience-dependent functional specialization of neural networks. In a pioneering series of postmortem histological studies of synaptic density in human cortex, Huttenlocher (1979, 1990) noted a general developmental pattern of initial overproduction of synapses followed by reductions to adult levels. For example, synaptic density in Layer III of the middle frontal gyrus reaches a peak at about 1 year of age that is considerably higher than the adult level, remains high until at least age 7 years, and then declines by about 40% until about age 16, when the adult level is finally attained.

Developmental neuroimaging research examining gray matter, which is comprised of neurons with dendritic and synaptic processes, as well as glia and vasculature, confirms that a prominent pattern seen in many cortical regions (especially dorsal regions) is that of increases in gray matter volume (or cortical thickness) in infancy and early childhood followed by gradual decreases that start in late childhood and continue into adulthood, when they plateau (e.g., Gogtay et al., 2004; Jernigan & Tallal, 1990; O'Donnell, Noseworthy, Levine, & Dennis, 2005; Pfefferbaum et al., 1994; Reiss, Abrams, Singer, Ross, & Denckla, 1996).

Reductions in gray matter during childhood have been attributed to synaptic pruning, which may occur in a Hebbian fashion, as a function of learning and experience (Casey, Giedd, & Thomas, 2000; Durston et al., 2001; Giedd et al., 1999), and which may result in the increasing differentiation of cognitive functions as neural regions become more specialized. A classic example of this process occurs in perceptual development. Initially, for example, occipital cortical areas involved in vision are activated by crossmodal input from other sensory modalities (reviewed in Collignon, Voss, Lassonde, & Lepore, 2009; Spector & Maurer, 2009). With normal visual experience, however, visual inputs to occipital cortex are reinforced whereas crossmodal inputs from other perceptual systems are eliminated or inhibited.

A similar process may occur more broadly in brain development, including in higher-order association areas that integrate information from lower-order, earlier developing areas such as visual cortex. According to one influential model, the Interactive Specialization model (e.g., Johnson & Munakata, 2005), neurocognitive development in general involves the increasing functional specialization of neural systems that are initially relatively undifferentiated but which become more specialized (or modularized) as part of a developmental process of adaption. Current research on executive function, for example, provides evidence that supports this suggestion. A seminal study of the factor structure of executive function in young adulthood used confirmatory factor analysis to extract three correlated latent variables from several commonly used executive function tasks, believed to represent cognitive flexibility, inhibitory control, and working memory (Miyake et al., 2000). Research with younger participants suggests that this differentiation of executive function into three dissociable components emerges during childhood. Among preschool-age children, research generally is consistent with a 1-factor solution (Wiebe, Espy, & Charak, 2008; Wiebe et al., 2011). Wiebe et al. (2008) used a battery of three tasks designed to measure working memory and seven tasks requiring inhibition, all of which loaded onto a single factor. This pattern was also found during the transition to adolescence (8–14 years) in a study by Prencipe et al. (2011). In contrast, several studies have found that the tripartite model of EF provides a good account of the data by middle childhood (Lehto, Juujärvi, Kooistra, & Pulkkinen, 2003; Visu-Petra, Benga, & Miclea, 2007), although Huizinga, Dolan, and van der Molen (2006) found that only working memory and shifting measures (and not inhibition measures) loaded onto latent variables in 7, 11, 15, and 21 year olds. In general, research on the factor structure of executive function appears to be consistent with a shift from diffuse to more focal cortical brain activity with age (Durston et al., 2006).

Evaluating Construct Validity in the NIH Toolbox CB

Convergent and discriminant validity are important elements of construct validity and relate to the dimensions accounting for covariance among groups of tests selected to measure specific domains. Construct validity is supported when (a) the empirically observed dimensions correspond to the a priori conceptual model for the domains being measured, and (b) individual tests are strongly related to the dimensions hypothesized from the conceptual model and are not related (or are more weakly related) to other dimensions. This process is somewhat more complicated in children due to the progressive differentiation of cognitive abilities that occurs as brain systems develop. In adults, a six-dimensional model of cognitive abilities should be appropriate to explain the relations among CB and validation measures, and it would be expected that CB measures of specific domains and corresponding validation measures would define dimensions that directly correspond to the six CB domains (see Weintraub et al., Chapter 1, this volume). In children, one would expect: (a) fewer dimensions underlying intercorrelations among tests, and (b) stronger associations among differentiable dimensions of the CB and the validation tests. In particular, executive function and working memory tasks would be expected to be less differentiated from other cognitive abilities, with lesser differentiation in younger children than in older children, because of the substantial development of frontal lobe structure and function that occurs throughout childhood and adolescence, continuing into early adulthood.

Data analyses related to this chapter were designed to test systematically how well alternative, a priori defined, dimensional models account for associations among NIHTB-CB and validation tests. Alternate models ranged from a simple 1-factor model representing a single global-cognition model to a 6-factor model corresponding to the six CB subdomains. It was hypothesized that CB and corresponding validation measures would define the same factors, but that fewer factors might be needed in children than in adults, and that intercorrelations among factors would be relatively high in children compared with adults. It was further hypothesized that age would be strongly related to all factors in children.

METHOD

Participants

In addition to the child and adolescent participants in the validation study (see Weintraub et al., Chapter 1, this volume; Table 3), we examined data from 267 adults (age 20–85 years, $M = 52.3$, $SD = 21.0$) in order to enhance model estimation for the 8- to 15-year-old age group.

Measures

CB and validation tests are listed in Table 14. Development of CB tests is described in detail in the chapters for each subdomain, and validation tests also are described in more detail in individual subdomain chapters.

TABLE 14

Measures and Associated Domains by Age Group

Age Group	Measure	Associated Domains
Both	**TPVT**	Vocabulary, Language, Crystallized/Global
	PPVT-IV	Vocabulary, Language, Crystallized/Global
	TORRT	Reading, Language, Crystallized, Global
	WRAT-R	Reading, Language, Crystallized, Global
	TPSMT	Episodic Memory, Fluid, Global
	TLSWMT	Working Memory, Fluid, Global
	TFIC + AT	Fluid, Global
	TDCCST	Fluid, Global
	TPCPST	Fluid, Global
3–6	WPPSI-III Block Design	Fluid, Global
	NEPSY-II Sentence Repetition	Episodic/Working Memory, Fluid, Global
8–15	PASAT	Working Memory, Fluid, Global
	Wechsler Letter Number Sorting	Working Memory, Fluid, Global
	Wechsler Digit Symbol	Speed, Executive/Speed, Fluid, Global
	Wechsler Symbol Search	Speed, Executive/Speed, Fluid, Global
	Wisconsin Card Sort Total Errors	Executive, Executive/Speed, Fluid, Global
	DKEFS Stroop Interference	Executive, Executive/Speed, Fluid, Global

Note. Domains are listed in order from most specific to most general. CB measures are bolded. TPVT, Toolbox Picture Vocabulary Test; PPVT-IV, Peabody Picture Vocabulary Test-4th Edition; TORRT, Toolbox Oral Reading Recognition Test; WRAT-R, Wide Range Reading Test-Revised; TPSMT, Toolbox Picture Sequence Memory Test; TLSWMT, Toolbox List Sorting Working Memory; TFIC + AT, Toolbox Flanker Inhibitory Control and Attention Test; TDCCST, Toolbox Dimensional Change Card Sort Test; TPCPST, Toolbox Pattern Comparison Processing Speed Test; WPPSI-III, Wechsler Preschool and Primary Intelligence Test; 3rd Edition; NEPSY-II, Developmental Neuropsychological Assessment, 2nd Edition; PASAT, Paced Auditory Serial Attention Test; DKEFS, Delis–Kaplan Executive Function Scales. © 2006–2013 National Institutes of Health and Northwestern University.

Data Analysis

Latent variable modeling methods were used to test convergent and discriminant validity of CB and validation measures. This process was performed separately in children aged 3–6 years and in the 8–15 year olds because different validation measures were administered to these two age groups due to a lack of established measures that are suitable across the entire age range. The basic process for both age groups was to perform a series of confirmatory factor analyses to test alternate models for the dimensions hypothesized to underlie the CB and validation tests. However, methodological limitations inherent in the design of the CB validation study led to differences in how analyses were performed.

The sample of children in the 3- to 6-year age range ($n = 119$) was sufficient to support the proposed analyses of their data, but this group received a smaller battery of tests. Consequently, not all domains had more than one observed indicator so fewer dimensions could be tested. The available sample for 8–15 year olds ($n = 88$) was relatively small for CFA purposes, but data for the same measures were available from the adults in the validation study, and these data were used to facilitate the analyses for 8–15 year olds. Specifically, the 8- to 15-year-old age group and adults ($n = 267$) were included in a multiple group CFA. In multiple group CFA modeling, a common model for both groups is specified on an a priori basis, and then group differences in individual parameters can be systematically tested. The advantage of this approach for the analysis of data from the older children is that many model parameters should be invariant across groups, and the combined sample size is used to estimate those parameters; this improves stability of estimates for the overall model. In effect, the results for the 8- to 15-year-old sample "borrow strength" from the adult sample through the use of invariance constraints on common parameter estimates, yielding a more stable pattern of results than would have occurred if the 8- to 15-year sample were analyzed separately. The focus for this study was on children and adolescents, however, so incorporation of adults when analyzing the older children data was primarily methodologically motivated. A subsequent report will address CB dimensions in adults.

The alternative models that were tested are shown in Table 15. Specific measures for each age group are presented in Table 14 along with their associated conceptual domains/dimensions in the various models. For the 3- to 6-year-old age group, the five models shown in Table 15 were separately estimated and model fit indices were compared to identify the best fitting model. The best fitting model at this stage had a simple structure with each indicator loading on just one factor. Modification indices were then examined to identify cross loadings of CB measures on other factors that would significantly improve model fit if freely estimated. Convergent validity

TABLE 15
Alternate Dimensional Models Underlying NIH Toolbox CB and Validation Measures

3–6 year olds	8–15 year olds
1f: Global Cognition	1f: Global Cognition
2f: Crystallized, Fluid	2f: Crystallized, Fluid
2f: Episodic/Working Memory, Nonmemory	2f: Memory, Nonmemory
3f: Crystallized, Fluid, Episodic/Working Memory	3f: Crystallized, Fluid, Memory
3f: Vocabulary, Reading, Fluid	3f: Language, Memory/Working Memory, Executive/Speed
4f: Vocabulary, Reading, Fluid, Episodic/Working Memory	3f: Language, Memory, Working Memory/Executive/Speed
	4f: Language, Memory, Working Memory, Executive/Speed
	4f: Vocabulary, Reading, Memory, Executive
	5f: Language, Memory, Working Memory, Executive, Speed
	5f: Vocabulary, Reading, Memory, Working Memory, Executive/Speed
	6f: Vocabulary, Reading, Memory, Working Memory, Executive, Speed

for a CB measure was evidenced by a strong loading on the dimension corresponding to the primary conceptual domain. Discriminant validity was shown if no loading, or a smaller loading, was required for a CB measure on a secondary dimension/domain.

Dimensional structure for the 8- to 15-year-old age group was evaluated using a multiple group CFA that included adults as the second group. The alternative dimensional models presented in Table 15 were estimated separately, the best fitting model was determined, and then cross loadings were tested. The basic process was similar to that for the 3- to 6-year age group, but the process for estimating each alternate model was different. First, a model was fitted with loadings and intercepts that were constrained to be equal in the two groups, but common factor means, variances, and covariances and unique factor variances for individual indicators were allowed to differ across groups. Then, modification indices were used to identify noninvariant loadings and then intercepts that subsequently were freely estimated in each group. This was an iterative process. The constrained loading with the largest modification index was freely estimated first, and then the constrained loading with the largest modification index from that analysis was freely estimated. This iterative process was continued until no additional significant modification indices for loadings were identified. The same process was then followed for intercepts. This process was continued to identify any additional loadings and then any additional intercepts. Fit indices from the different alternative models at this stage of development were compared in order to identify the best fitting model. After a best fitting model was chosen, further modification to that model was achieved by including residual correlations that were conceptually justified and improved model fit in both groups. Finally, modification indices were used to identify significant cross-loadings of Toolbox measures on secondary factors.

Variables were recoded prior to analysis using the Blom rank order normalization algorithm in SAS Proc Rank. This resulted in variables with relatively normal distributions and also established a common scale of measurement of all variables. The normalization was applied separately to the 3- to 6-year-old group and the combined 8- to 15-year-old and adult groups. Scores for DKEFS Stroop Interference and Wisconsin Card Sort Total Errors were inverted so that higher scores indicated better performance on all measures. Normalized scores were multiplied by 3.0 and added to 10.0 to place them on a common scale with mean of 10.0 and standard deviation of 3.0.

Model estimation was performed with Mplus version 6.0 (Muthén & Muthén, 1998–2010) using a maximum likelihood estimator for continuous variables applied to a mean and covariance data structure. Latent variable modeling traditionally uses an overall chi square test of model fit, often supplemented by a number of fit indices to better characterize model fit. Commonly used fit indices include the comparative fit index (CFI; Bentler, 1990), the Tucker-Lewis index (TLI; Tucker & Lewis, 1973), the root mean square error of approximation (RMSEA; Browne & Cudek, 1993), and the standardized root mean squared residual (SRMR; Bentler, 1995). The chi-square difference test (Steiger, Shapiro, & Browne, 1985) was used to determine if fit significantly improved as a result of freeing one or more parameters in a model. Modification indices correspond to the improvement in model fit as measured by the amount the overall chi square value would decrease if a constrained parameter were freely estimated. A threshold of 6.63 was used as a standard for significant improvement in fit, which corresponds to $p = .01$ for a chi square variate with 1 degree of freedom.

RESULTS

Children 3–6 Years of Age

A 3-factor model (Vocabulary, Reading, Fluid abilities) was the best fitting of the alternate models and showed relatively good absolute fit on all indices except RMSEA (see Table 16). Fit for this 3-factor model was substantially better than either the 2-factor model or the 1-factor model. There were

TABLE 16
Fit Indices for Alternate Models of Cognitive Dimensions in 3–6 Year Olds and 8–15 Year Olds

Model	Overall χ^2 [df]	χ^2: 8–15	CFI	TLI	RMSEA (90% CI)	SRMR
3–6 Year Age Group						
1f: Global	214.1 [44]		.824	.780	.180 (.156–.205)	.057
2f: Crystallized, Fluid	168.3 [43]		.870	.834	.156 (.132–.182)	.090
2f: Episodic/Working Memory, Nonmemory	214.1 [43]		.823	.773	.183 (.159–.208)	.057
3f: Vocabulary, Reading, Fluid	76.8 [41]		.963	.950	.086 (.055–.115)	.039
8–15 Year Age Group						
1f: Global	1278.0 [241]	248.0	.725	.689	.156 (.147–.164)	.081
2f: Crystallized, Fluid	607.6 [245]	215.8	.904	.893	.091 (.082–.100)	.119
2f: Episodic/Working Memory, Nonmemory						
3f: Language, Episodic/Working Memory, Working Memory/Executive	734.9 [250]	251.2	.871	.860	.105 (.053–.113)	.106
3f: Vocabulary, Reading, Fluid	477.8 [241]	172.7	.937	.929	.074 (.053–.074)	.079
4f: Vocabulary, Reading, Memory, Working Memory/Executive	412.8 [239]	170.6	.954	.947	.064 (.065–.084)	.109
4f: Vocabulary, Reading, Episodic/Working Memory, Executive	456.7 [239]	176.0	.942	.934	.072 (.062–.082)	.103
5f: Vocabulary, Reading, Episodic Memory, Working Memory, Executive	370.5 [230]	162.3	.963	.956	.059 (.047–.069)	.109

Note. χ^2: 8–15 shows the specific contribution of the 8- to 15-year-old group to the overall χ^2-value; CFI = comparative fit index; TLI = Tucker-Lewis index; CI = confidence interval; RMSEA = root mean square error of approximation.

TABLE 17

STANDARDIZED FACTOR LOADINGS (STANDARD ERRORS IN PARENTHESES) FOR BEST FITTING 3-FACTOR MODEL FOR 3- to 6-YEAR-OLD AGE GROUP

Latent Factor	Observed Indicator	Loading
Reading	**TORRT**	.97 (.02)
	WRAT-R	.96 (.02)
Vocabulary	**TPVT**	.75 (.05)
	PPVT-IV	.99 (.03)
Fluid Abilities	**TPSMT**	.79 (.04)
	TLSWMT	.70 (.05)
	TFIC + AT	.83 (.04)
	TDCCST	.89 (.03)
	TPCPST	.70 (.06)
	NEPSY-II Sentence Repetition	.78 (.04)
	WPPSI-III Block Design	.77 (.04)

Note. CB measures are bolded. Correlation of Reading with Vocabulary = .69 ($SE = .06$, $p < .001$), Reading with Fluid Abilities = .83 ($SE = .04$, $p < .001$), Vocabuary with Fluid Abilities = .83 ($SE = .04$, $p < .001$). TORRT, Toolbox Oral Reading Recognition Test; WRAT-R, Wide Range Reading Test: Revised; TPVT, Toolbox Picture Vocabulary Test; PPVT-IV, Peabody Picture Vocabulary Test: 4th Edition; TPSMT, Toolbox Picture Sequence Memory Test; TLSWMT, Toolbox List Sorting Working Memory; TFIC + AT, Toolbox Flanker Inhibitory Control and Attention Test; TDCCST, Toolbox Dimensional Change Card Sort Test; TPCPST, Toolbox Pattern Comparison Processing Speed Test; NEPSY-II, Developmental Neuropsychological Assessment, 2nd Edition; WPPSI-III, Wechsler Preschool and Primary Intelligence Test, 3rd Edition.

estimation problems for the 3-factor and 4-factor models that had separate dimensions for memory and fluid abilities because the correlation of the memory and fluid abilities latent variables were indistinguishable from 1.0.

Standardized loadings for the best fitting model are presented in Table 17. Factor loadings were strong for all factors and indicators. None of the CB measures had significant loadings on secondary factors. The correlation of the Reading and Vocabulary factors was .68 ($SE = .06$, $p < .001$), and the correlations of Fluid Abilities with Reading and Vocabulary were both .83 ($SEs = .04$, $ps < .001$). These results indicate that reading and vocabulary are clearly differentiated from other cognitive abilities and from each other in this age group, but other cognitive abilities are not well differentiated. Results support the convergent and discriminant validity of the Toolbox reading and vocabulary measures and indicate that the other CB tests measure fluid ability that is not well differentiated in children in this age range. Within this range, however, all three factors were highly correlated with age: Reading, $r = .75$ ($SE = .04$, $p < .001$), Vocabulary, $r = .67$ ($SE = .05$, $p < .001$), and Fluid Abilities, $r = .86$ ($SE = .03$, $p < .001$).

Children 8–15 Years of Age

A 5-factor model (Vocabulary, Reading, Episodic Memory, Working Memory, Executive/Speed) was identified as the best fitting model for the sample of 8–15 year olds (see Table 16). Estimation problems arose for the 6-factor model in the 8- to 15-year age group due to the correlation between the Executive and Speed factors being close to 1.0. (The 6-factor model provided the best fit for adults, not shown.) Model fit for the best fitting 5-factor model was good after accounting for noninvariant parameters across the two groups and including modifications to estimate covariances among unique factors for measures that overlap in methods (Wechsler Digit Symbol and Symbol Search; Toolbox Flanker Inhibitory Control and Attention Test, Toolbox DCCS, and Toolbox Pattern Comparison Processing Speed Test). The Toolbox List Sorting Working Memory Test had a significant cross loading on the Episodic Memory factor in the 8- to 15-year age group, but no other significant cross-loadings of CB variables on secondary factors were found.

Six variables had noninvariant loadings. DKEFS Stroop Interference was a stronger indicator of Executive/Speed in the 8–15 year olds than in adults (standardized loadings of .90 vs. .80), and Wechsler Letter Number Sorting and PASAT were stronger indicators of Working Memory in 8–15 year olds (.82 vs. .66 and .91 vs. .75). The Toolbox Picture Sequence Memory Test was less strongly related to Episodic Memory in the 8- to 15-year-old group (.68 vs. .81). The Toolbox Picture Vocabulary Test was less strongly related to the Vocabulary factor, and Digit Symbol was more strongly related to Executive/Speed in the 8–15 year olds, but the standardized loadings were minimally different (.85 vs. .91 and .82 vs. .77). Six variables had noninvariant intercepts; Wechsler Digit Symbol and PASAT were relatively easier in adults, and the Toolbox Picture Sequence Memory Test, Toolbox DCCS, WCST Errors, Toolbox Flanker and the Toolbox Pattern Comparison Processing Speed Test were relatively easier in the 8–15 year olds. That is, the expected performance for the latter five variables was better in the children than in adults after equating for the latent ability measured by the relevant factors.

Standardized loadings for the best fitting model are presented in Table 18. Loadings for the Toolbox Oral Reading Recognition Test and the Toolbox Picture Vocabulary Test were quite strong, ranging from .85 to .98. The Toolbox Picture Sequence Memory Test had a standardized loading of .68 on the Episodic Memory factor and the Toolbox DCCS had a loading of .71 on the Executive/Speed factor. The Toolbox Flanker and the Toolbox Pattern Comparison Processing Speed Test had loadings on the Executive/Speed factor in the .55–.60 range and the Toolbox List Sorting Working Memory Test had a loading of .54 on the Working Memory factor. Toolbox List Sorting had a secondary loading of .29 on the Episodic Memory factor. Overall, these findings show evidence of excellent convergent validity. The presence of only one, relatively weak cross loading supports discriminant validity of the CB. The weakest convergent validity estimates were for the CB measures of Executive/Speed, and this is not surprising because of the relative heterogeneity of the indicators for this factor and the absence of

TABLE 18

STANDARDIZED FACTOR LOADINGS (STANDARD ERRORS IN PARENTHESES) FOR BEST FITTING 5-FACTOR MODEL FOR 8–15 YEAR OLDS

Latent Factor	Observed Indicator	Loading
Reading	**TORRT**	.98 (.01)
	WRAT-R	.96 (.01)
Vocabulary	**TPVT**	.86 (.03)
	PPVT-IV	.97 (.02)
Episodic Memory	**TPSMT**	.68 (.08)
	RAVLT	.70 (.04)
	BVMT	.78 (.04)
	TLSWMT[a]	.29 (.07)
Working Memory	**TLSWMT**	.54 (.04)
	PASAT	.82 (.04)
	Wechsler Letter Number Sorting	.91 (.03)
Executive/Speed	**TFIC + AT**	.59 (.04)
	TDCCST	.71 (.04)
	TPCPST	.58 (.04)
	Wechsler Digit Symbol	.82 (.04)
	Wechsler Symbol Search	.74 (.03)
	Wisconsin Card Sort Total Errors	.69 (.04)
	D-KEFS Stroop Interference	.90 (.03)

Note. CB Measures are bolded. TORRT, Toolbox Oral Reading Recognition Test; WRAT-R, Wide Range Reading Test-Revised; TPVT, Toolbox Picture Vocabulary Test; PPVT-IV, Peabody Picture Vocabulary Test-4th Edition; TPSMT, Toolbox Picture Sequence Memory Test; BVMT-R: Brief Visuospatial Memory Test-Revised; RAVLT, Rey Auditory Verbal Learning Test; TLSWMT, Toolbox List Sorting Working Memory; PASAT, Paced Auditory Serial Attention Test; TFIC + AT, Toolbox Flanker Inhibitory Control and Attention Test; TDCCST, Toolbox Dimensional Change Card Sort Test; TPCPST, Toolbox Pattern Comparison Processing Speed Test; D-KEFS, Delis-Kaplan Executive Function Scales.
[a]Significant loading on secondary factor.

direct analogues of the Toolbox measures as were available for the Toolbox Oral Reading Recognition Test and the Toolbox Picture Vocabulary Test.

The intercorrelations of the five factors for the 8–15 year olds were very high, ranging from .72 to .94 ($ps < .001$, see Table 19). Whereas the abilities

TABLE 19

INTER-CORRELATION OF FACTORS FROM BEST-FITTING 5-FACTOR MODEL FOR 8–15 YEAR OLDS

	Reading	Vocabulary	Episodic Memory	Working Memory
Vocabulary	.89 (.03)			
Episodic Memory	.72 (.07)	.85 (.06)		
Working Memory	.87 (.04)	.83 (.04)	.90 (.06)	
Executive/Speed	.91 (.03)	.90 (.03)	.89 (.06)	.94 (.03)

Note. Standard errors in parentheses ($p < .001$ for all correlations).

TABLE 20
INTER-CORRELATION OF FACTORS FROM BEST-FITTING 5-FACTOR MODEL FOR ADULTS

	Reading	Vocabulary	Episodic Memory	Working Memory
Vocabulary	.82 (.03)			
Episodic Memory	.30 (.06)	.12 (.07)		
Working Memory	.54 (.05)	.43 (.06)	.84 (.04)	
Executive/Speed	.41 (.06)	.23 (.07)	.80 (.04)	.90 (.03)

Note. Standard errors in parentheses ($p < .001$ for all correlations except Vocabulary with Episodic Memory, where $p = .07$). © 2006–2013 National Institutes of Health and Northwestern University.

being measured by these factors were differentiable, they nevertheless were highly correlated, which is likely due to broad differences in overall development within this age group that contribute substantial, nonspecific influences on cognitive function. For comparison purposes, factor correlations for the Adult group are presented in Table 20. Correlations of the Toolbox Oral Reading Recognition Test and the Toolbox Picture Vocabulary Test with Episodic Memory, Working Memory, and Executive/Speed factors were substantially smaller. Correlations among the latter three factors were still quite high, but were smaller than were observed in the 8–15 year olds. All five factors were highly correlated with age: Reading, $r = .70$ ($SE = .05$, $p < .001$); Vocabulary, $r = .76$ ($SE = .06$, $p < .001$); Episodic Memory, $r = .53$ ($SE = .10$, $p < .001$); Working Memory, $r = .64$ ($SE = .08$, $p < .001$); and Executive/Speed, $r = .86$ ($SE = .04$, $p < .001$).

DISCUSSION

There were four primary findings from this study. First, CB measures and their corresponding validation measures consistently defined common factors in a pattern that broadly supported the convergent and discriminant validity of the CB. Second, we found fewer empirically distinct dimensions in children in the 8- to 15-year age range than in adults, and still fewer distinct dimensions in the 3–6 year olds. In the 8–15 age range, executive function and processing speed were less differentiated than in adults, and in the 3–6 year olds, measures of episodic memory, working memory, executive function, and speed all defined a common fluid abilities dimension. Third, correlations among identified dimensions were stronger in children than in adults, and this was especially evident in much stronger correlations in children of crystallized abilities (vocabulary and reading) with other abilities. Fourth, age was strongly related to the cognitive dimensions underlying test performance.

Three distinct dimensions were identified for the 3–6 years age group: vocabulary, reading, and fluid abilities. CB measures were strong indicators of these dimensions and no significant cross-loadings on secondary dimensions were found. These results support the convergent and discriminant validity of the CB measures in this age range, but suggest that the full 6-subdomain model that guided test development is less applicable in this age range because fluid abilities are not well differentiated.

Five separable dimensions were found in the 8–15 year olds. These dimensions corresponded to the subdomains in the test development model for the CB measures with the exception that Executive Function and Processing Speed were not clearly separable. The five dimensions that were observed in this age range were highly correlated, likely reflecting the broad impact of age, experience, and associated brain development in this group.

A striking and somewhat unexpected outcome was the finding that reading and vocabulary were clearly separable in both the 3–6 and 8–15 age groups. Model fit was consistently higher in both groups when vocabulary and reading measures defined separate factors as opposed to a common language or crystallized abilities factor. Although reading and vocabulary were highly correlated in both groups, they nevertheless defined distinct dimensions and were less correlated with one another than were dimensions underlying fluid abilities.

All latent factors identified in both the 3- to 6- and 8- to 15-year-old age groups were substantially correlated with age, with correlations ranging from .53 to .86. The Fluid Abilities factor in the 3–6 year olds and the Executive/Speed factor in the 8–15 year olds were very highly correlated with age. These results likely show the profound influences of brain development coupled with life experiences on cognitive abilities. The sensitivity to age suggests that the Toolbox CB will be useful for tracking cognitive development in longitudinal studies in children.

This study had a number of limitations. The sample size was relatively small for confirmatory factor analysis, and fewer and different tests were administered to the 3- to 6-year-old group. Consequently, we could not incorporate both the 3- to 6- and the 8- to 15-year-old age groups into a combined analysis. The issue of measurement invariance at different ages is especially important for the intended use of the NIH Toolbox. Being able to measure cognition on a common metric across the entire age span from 3 years to late adulthood is an important goal for the CB, and formal testing of factorial invariance in different age groups is required to show a common metric. The multiple group analysis of 8–15 year olds and adults constituted a preliminarily examination of measurement invariance. Groups sizes in the 3- to 6-year and 8- to-15-year age groups were relatively small, which likely affects stability of results, and consequently, any conclusions about measurement invariance must be considered tentative. The norming study (projected $N = 4,000$) for the Toolbox will offer a unique opportunity to formally test measurement invariance with much larger samples across the full age range from age 3 years to the end of life. The norming sample will also include a sizeable group of individuals tested in Spanish ($N = 500$) and this will provide an opportunity for evaluating measurement variance across the English and Spanish versions of the battery.

In spite of these limitations, these results show favorable evidence for the construct validity of the NIH Toolbox CB across early and mid childhood and adolesence and demonstrate how this battery can be useful for understanding the evolving structure of cognition over the course of development. Having standardized methods available for assessing cognition across the lifespan along with the other domains measured by the NIH Toolbox including emotion, motor functioning, and sensory functioning will provide an important resource for research to further our understanding of brain and cognitive development.

REFERENCES

Bentler, P. M. (1990). Comparative fit indices in structural models. *Psychological Bulletin*, **107**, 238–246.

Bentler, P. M. (1995). *EQS structural equations program manual.* Encino, CA: Multivariate Software.

Browne, M., & Cudek, R. (1993). Alternate ways of assessing model fit. In K. Bollen & J. Long (Eds.), *Testing structural equation models* (pp. 136–162). Thousand Oaks, CA: SAGE.

Casey, B. J., Giedd, J. N., & Thomas, K. M. (2000). Structural and functional brain development and its relation to cognitive development. *Biological Psychology*, **54**(1–3), 241–257.

Collignon, O., Voss, P., Lassonde, M., & Lepore, F. (2009). Cross-modal plasticity for the spatial processing of sounds in visually deprived subjects. *Experimental Brain Research*, **192**(3), 343–358.

Durston, S., Davidson, M. C., Tottenham, N., Galvan, A., Spicer, J., Fossella, J. A., et al. (2006). A shift from diffuse to focal cortical activity with development. *Developmental Science*, **9**(1), 1–8.

Durston, S., Hulshoff Pol, H. E., Casey, B. J., Giedd, J. N., Buitelaar, J. K., & van Engeland, H. (2001). Anatomical MRI of the developing human brain: What have we learned? *Journal of the American Academy of Child and Adolescent Psychiatry*, **40**(9), 1012–1020.

Giedd, J. N., Blumenthal, J., Jeffries, N. O., Castellanos, F. X., Liu, H., Zijdenbos, A., et al. (1999). Brain development during childhood and adolescence: A longitudinal MRI study. *Nature Neuroscience*, **2**(10), 861–863.

Gogtay, N., Giedd, J. N., Lusk, L., Hayashi, K. M., Greenstein, D., Vaituzis, A. C., et al. (2004). Dynamic mapping of human cortical development during childhood through early adulthood. *Proceedings of the National Academy of Sciences United States of America*, **101**(21), 8174–8179.

Huizinga, M. T., Dolan, C. V., & van der Molen, M. W. (2006). Age-related change in executive function: Developmental trends and a latent variable analysis. *Neuropsychologia (Special Issue: Advances in Developmental Cognitive Neuroscience)*, **44**(11), 2017–2036.

Huttenlocher, P. R. (1979). Synaptic density in human frontal cortex—Developmental changes and effects of aging. *Brain Research*, **163**(2), 195–205.

Huttenlocher, P. R. (1990). Morphometric study of human cerebral cortex development. *Neuropsychologia*, **28**(6), 517–527.

Jernigan, T. L., & Tallal, P. (1990). Late childhood changes in brain morphology observable with MRI. *Developmental Medicine and Child Neurology*, **32**(5), 379–385.

Johnson, M. H., & Munakata, Y. (2005). Processes of change in brain and cognitive development. *Trends in Cognitive Sciences*, **9**(3), 152–158.

Lehto, J. E., Juujärvi, P., Kooistra, L., & Pulkkinen, L. (2003). Dimensions of executive functioning: Evidence from children. *British Journal of Developmental Psychology*, **21**(1), 59–80.

Miyake, A., Friedman, N. P., Emerson, M. J., Witzki, A. H., Howerter, A., & Wager, T. D. (2000). The unity and diversity of executive functions and their contributions to complex "Frontal Lobe" tasks: A latent variable analysis. *Cognitive Psychology*, **41**(1), 49–100.

Muthén, L. K., & Muthén, B. O. (1998–2010). *Mplus User's Guide* (6th ed.). Los Angeles, CA: Muthén & Muthén.

O'Donnell, S., Noseworthy, M. D., Levine, B., & Dennis, M. (2005). Cortical thickness of the frontopolar area in typically developing children and adolescents. *NeuroImage*, **24**(4), 948–954.

Pfefferbaum, A., Mathalon, D. H., Sullivan, E. V., Rawles, J. M., Zipursky, R. B., & Lim, K. O. (1994). A quantitative magnetic resonance imaging study of changes in brain morphology from infancy to late adulthood. *Archives of Neurology*, **51**(9), 874–887.

Prencipe, A., Kesek, A., Cohen, J., Lamm, C., Lewis, M. D., & Zelazo, P. D. (2011). Development of hot and cool executive function during the transition to adolescence. *Journal of Experimental Child Psychology*, **108**(3), 621–637.

Reiss, A. L., Abrams, M. T., Singer, H. S., Ross, J. L., & Denckla, M. B. (1996). Brain development, gender and IQ in children: A volumetric imaging study. *Brain*, **119**(Pt 5), 1763–1774.

Spector, F., & Maurer, D. (2009). Synesthesia: A new approach to understanding the development of perception. *Developmental Psychology*, **45**(1), 175–189.

Steiger, J. H., Shapiro, A., & Browne, M. W. (1985). On the multivariate asymptotic distribution of sequential chi-square statistics. *Psychometrika*, **50**, 253–264.

Tucker, L. R., & Lewis, C. (1973). A reliability coefficient for maximum likelihood factor analysis. *Psychometrika*, **38**, 1–10.

Visu-Petra, L., Benga, O., & Miclea, M. (2007). Dimensions of attention and executive functioning in 5- to 12-year-old children: Neuropsychological assessment with the NEPSY battery. *Cognition, Brain, Behavior (Special Issue: Developmental Cognitive Neuropsychology)*, **11**(3), 585–608.

Wiebe, S. A., Espy, K. A., & Charak, D. (2008). Using confirmatory factor analysis to understand executive control in preschool children: I. Latent structure. *Developmental Psychology*, **44**(2), 575–587.

Wiebe, S. A., Sheffield, T., Nelson, J. M., Clark, C. A., Chevalier, N., & Espy, K. A. (2011). The structure of executive function in 3-year-olds. *Journal of Experimental Child Psychology*, **108**(3), 436–452.

VIII. NIH TOOLBOX COGNITION BATTERY (CB): COMPOSITE SCORES OF CRYSTALLIZED, FLUID, AND OVERALL COGNITION

Natacha Akshoomoff, Jennifer L. Beaumont, Patricia J. Bauer,
Sureyya S. Dikmen, Richard C. Gershon, Dan Mungas, Jerry Slotkin,
David Tulsky, Sandra Weintraub, Philip David Zelazo, and Robert K. Heaton

ABSTRACT The NIH Toolbox Cognition Battery (CB) includes 7 tests covering 6 cognitive abilities. This chapter describes the psychometric characteristics in children ages 3–15 years of a total summary score and composite scores reflecting two major types of cognition: "crystallized" (more dependent upon past learning experiences) and "fluid" (capacity for new learning and information processing in novel situations). Both types of cognition are considered important in everyday functioning, but are thought to be differently affected by brain health status throughout life, from early childhood through older adulthood. All three Toolbox composite scores showed excellent test–retest reliability, robust developmental effects across the childhood age range considered here, and strong correlations with established measures of similar abilities. Additional preliminary evidence of validity includes significant associations between all three Toolbox composite scores and maternal reports of children's health status and school performance.

The NIH Toolbox Cognition Battery (CB) is comprised of 7 test instruments that are described in detail in Chapters 2–6 of this monograph. Many researchers will want to consider these measures separately, but others are expected to focus on a smaller number of composite scores that represent overall cognition and/or certain categories of abilities. Such composite scores can be defined using factor analytic methods (see Mungas et al., Chapter 7, this volume) but these may yield different combinations of scores for different age groups and consequently may not be well suited to longitudinal research or research that spans multiple age ranges (e.g., early childhood to adult).

Corresponding author: Robert K. Heaton, Department of Psychiatry, 9500 Gilman Drive, University of California, San Diego, La Jolla, CA, 92093-0603, email: rheaton@ucsd.edu

Another approach to defining composite scores is to group tests that may tap more than one specific ability domain but share certain theoretical and psychometric characteristics across the lifespan. In the two-component theory of intellectual development (Cattell, 1971; Horn, 1968; 1970), for example, the premise is that the organization of *fluid* and *crystallized* abilities is dynamic, developing and transforming throughout the life span (Li et al., 2004). Fluid abilities are used to solve problems, think and act quickly, and encode new episodic memories, and play an important role in adapting to novel situations in everyday life. These abilities improve rapidly during childhood, typically reaching their peak in early adulthood, and then decline as adults get older. Crystallized abilities, in contrast, are presumed to be more dependent on experience. They represent an accumulation of verbal knowledge and skills, and thus are more heavily influenced by education and cultural exposure, particularly during childhood. These abilities show marked developmental change during childhood, but they typically continue to improve slightly into middle adulthood and then remain relatively stable.

Age-related improvements in fluid abilities in early development are thought to support acquisition of the knowledge needed for crystallized abilities, thus accounting for stronger correlations between fluid and crystallized abilities early in life, compared with those found in later years (Cattell, 1971; Horn, 1968). Once developed, crystallized abilities tend to be fairly stable throughout adulthood and much less susceptible to the effects of aging and health status during aging than is the case with fluid abilities. In contrast, fluid abilities tend to be more sensitive to neurobiological integrity, including changes in brain functioning with aging and in a variety of neurological disorders that alter brain structure and function.

Here we present data from the children's validation sample ($N = 208$) for the CB that is based on three candidate summary scores: Toolbox Crystallized Cognition Composite, Toolbox Fluid Cognition Composite, and Toolbox Cognitive Function Composite (a combination of both crystallized and fluid scores). We expected all three summary scores to increase fairly rapidly with age, in contrast to results obtained during adulthood (Weintraub et al., 2013). We also present psychometric information, such as test/retest reliability and associations with well accepted, but mostly proprietary, instruments that also putatively tap crystallized and fluid abilities (i.e., validation measures). Although we predicted that the CB summary scores would show excellent convergent validity with relevant validation measures, we expected that there would be less evidence of discriminant validity across fluid and crystallized abilities, particularly among younger children. This hypothesis was based upon the expectation that fluid and crystallized abilities develop rapidly and roughly in parallel during early childhood, whereas they tend to diverge during adulthood with larger age effects on fluid abilities

(Horn & Cattell, 1967; Sattler, 2001; Weintraub et al., 2013; WAIS-III WMS-III Technical Manual, 1997).

With both children and adults it is important to evaluate the potential impact of demographic variables on various neuropsychological tests (Heaton, Taylor, & Manly, 2003). For example, information about which demographic variables are associated with performance in healthy individuals can inform important group matching decisions in future research, as well as the creation and use of standards for evaluating performance relative to norms. In addition to predicted changes with age, performance on certain measures may also differ with respect to gender, family income, and race/ethnicity. Whereas level of formal education also is a significant predictor of cognitive test performance in adulthood (e.g., Heaton et al., 2003, 2004), in children age and education are almost totally confounded. However, for children, maternal level of education also has been shown to be a significant predictor of IQ and various aspects of neuropsychological test performance. The relation of each of these demographic variables with the composite measures of CB performance was examined.

Finally, to further explore validity of the Toolbox composite measures, we examined associations between all cognitive summary scores and a few relatively gross measures of health and everyday functioning (maternal reports of health and school performance).

METHOD

Participants

The sample on which the analyses are based is described in detail in Weintraub et al. (Chapter 1, this volume; Table 3). Additional demographic, health status and school functioning variables were based on the categorical information obtained from each participant's parent (typically, the mother). Family income was categorized into five levels (<$20,000 [11%], $20,000 to $39,999 [19%], $40,000 to $74,999 [34%], $75,000 to $99,999 [19%], and ≥$100,000 [16%]). Child health status was categorized as Excellent (69%) or Poor to Very Good (31%). For school age children (age 8–15), maternal ratings of academic performance were classified as Above Average (55%) or Below Average to Average (45%); also 19% of these children were reported to have required special (remedial) classes and/or tutoring in school.

NIH Toolbox CB Measures

The battery of seven CB tests included two measures of crystallized abilities (the Picture Vocabulary Test and the Oral Reading Recognition

Test), as well as six measures of fluid abilities (the Toolbox Dimensional Change Card Sort [DCCS] Test, the Toolbox Flanker Inhibitory Control and Attention Test, the Toolbox Picture Sequence Memory Test, the Toolbox List Sorting Working Memory Test, and the Toolbox Pattern Comparison Processing Speed Test). Descriptions of the individual CB tests and the derived scores that reflect the multiple domains of cognitive functioning are provided in Chapters 2–6 of this monograph. Raw scores from the CB measures were converted to normally distributed standard scores (scaled scores) having a mean of 10 and a standard deviation of 3. These standard scores were then averaged to compute the Toolbox Crystallized Cognition Composite, Toolbox Fluid Cognition Composite, and Toolbox Cognitive Function (i.e., Total) Composite scores. Three additional summary scores were computed in order to evaluate the use of a potential abbreviated version of the CB with children ages 3 to 6 years. Each abbreviated version included a subset of the tasks in the full battery. The three abbreviated versions were the (1) Short Toolbox Crystallized Cognition Score, which included only the Picture Vocabulary Test; (2) Short Toolbox Fluid Cognition Score, which included the Flanker Inhibitory Control and Attention Test and the Picture Sequence Memory Test, and (3) Short Toolbox Total Composite, which was a combination of the abbreviated crystallized and fluid scores.

Validation Measures

In Chapter 1, Tables 3 and 4 show the CB instruments and corresponding validation measures for each. Normalized standard scores (scaled scores) from two published and widely used measures, the Reading subtest from the Wide Range Achievement Test-4th Edition (Wilkinson & Robertson, 2006) and the Peabody Picture Vocabulary Test-4th Edition (PPVT-IV; Dunn & Dunn, 2007), were combined for the Validation Crystallized Composite score. Data available from validation fluid cognition measures varied with participants' age, because we are unaware of any previously published instruments that have been standardized for the full age range designated for the NIH Toolbox. In order to compare the CB Fluid Composite with validation measures for children ages 3–6 years, scaled scores from the Wechsler Preschool and Primary Scale of Intelligence-3rd Edition Block Design (Wechsler, 2002) and Sentence Repetition from the Developmental Neuropsychological Assessment, 2nd Edition (NEPSY-II; Korkman, Kirk, & Kemp, 2007) were combined for the Validation Fluid Composite score. For children ages 8–15, the Validation Fluid Composite score was derived from normalized scaled scores from the Wechsler Intelligence Scale for Children-4th Edition (WISC-IV) Letter-Number Sequencing subtest (Wechsler, 2003), an average of scores from the WISC-IV Coding and Symbol Search subtests (Wechsler, 2003), the Delis–Kaplan Executive Function System (Delis,

Kramer, & Kaplan, 2001) Color-Word Interference score, an average of total learning scores from the Brief Visuospatial Memory Test-Revised (Benedict, 1997) and the Rey Auditory Verbal Learning Test (Rey, 1964), and the Paced Auditory Serial Addition Test (Gronwall, 1977; first channel only). In order to evaluate the Short Toolbox scores for the 3 to 6 year olds, the Short Validation Crystallized score was based on the PPVT-IV score. Also for 3 to 6 year olds, Validation Fluid scores (combination of WPPSI-III Block Design and NEPSY-II Sentence Repetition) were compared with Short Toolbox Fluid Cognition scores.

Analyses

Nonage-adjusted, normalized scaled scores were computed for each CB measure. These were then averaged together to create normalized, composite scaled scores. Using data from the subset of participants for whom we had both test and retest data ($n = 66$, including $n = 38$ for ages 3–6 years and $n = 28$ for ages 8–15 years), Pearson correlations were computed to estimate test–retest reliability for the total retested group and for the age subgroups (3–6 years; 8–15 years) separately. The relation between each of the nonage-adjusted composite scores and age (in years) was then examined using data from the full sample of 208 children. Analyses of variance (ANOVAs) were then performed to examine other demographic associations with performance across each age-adjusted composite measure. Also, age-adjusted composite scores were examined for association with health and school functioning variables. Effect sizes are reported as Cohen's d, with cutoffs of .20, .50, and .80 indicating small, medium, and large effects, respectively.

Similarly, normalized composite scaled scores were constructed for the validation measures, and associations between corresponding CB and validation composite scores were computed. These had to be done separately for younger (ages 3–6 years) and older (8–15 years) children because the validation fluid measures were different for these age groups. Finally, again for the separate age groups, other psychometric properties of the CB and validation composite scores were compared.

RESULTS

Test–Retest Reliability

For the 66 participants across all ages (3–15 years) who were retested, excellent test-retest correlations were observed: $rs = .92$, .95, and .96 for Toolbox Crystallized, Fluid, and Total composite scores, respectively; all $df = 64$ and $ps < .0001$. The 3- to 6-year-old subgroup with longitudinal data ($n = 38$) also evidenced good test–retest correlations on the full Toolbox composite scores ($rs = .74$, .86, and .89 for Toolbox Crystallized, Fluid, and

Total, $df = 36$, $ps < .0001$). Their reliability estimates for the Short Fluid and Short Total composite scores were also acceptable ($rs = .78$ and $.73$, $df = 36$, $p < .0001$), although reliability of the Short Crystallized score (Picture Vocabulary only) was more modest ($r(36) = .50$, $p = .002$). The 28 participants aged 8–15 years who were retested obtained robust reliability estimates on the full composite scores, although these were somewhat lower than those seen with the total child group ($rs = .85$, $.76$, and $.88$ for Crystallized, Fluid, and Total, $df = 26$, $ps < .0001$).

"Practice effects" were computed as the means and standard deviations of the difference between the retest composite scaled score and the test composite scaled score, with significance of the effect being tested with t tests for dependent means. For the total child group (ages 3–15 years, $n = 66$), the Toolbox Crystallized Composite evidenced virtually no practice effect over an average two week test–retest interval: *mean practice effect* $= .00$, $SD = 1.18$, $t(65) = -.03$, $p = .98$. However, the Toolbox Fluid Composite score showed a significant effect of about a half of a scaled score point (*mean* $= .50$, $SD = .96$, $t(65) = 4.27$, $ES = .52$, $p < .0001$), and the Toolbox Total Composite also had a modest practice effect (*mean* $= .27$, $SD = .87$, $t(65) = 2.57$, $ES = .31$, $p = .01$). Interestingly, degree of practice effect was not significantly correlated with age for any of the Toolbox composite scores (Crystallized $r = .14$, Fluid $r = .06$, Total $r = .16$, $df = 64$, all $ps > .19$).

Age Effects

Pearson correlation coefficients were used to examine the relation between age and performance on the Toolbox composite measures. As shown in Figure 13, there was clear evidence that the Toolbox composite measures are sensitive to developmental growth during childhood. Across the 3- to 15-year age span ($N = 208$), age was highly correlated with performance on the Toolbox Crystallized Composite ($r(203) = .87$), Toolbox Fluid Composite ($r(205) = .86$), and Toolbox Total Composite ($r(205) = .88$) (all $ps < .0001$). Furthermore, Figure 13 shows almost overlapping, linear effects of age on the Toolbox Crystallized and Fluid Composite scores across the full age span from 3 to 15 years. It is noted as well that in this total child group the correlation between Crystallized and Fluid Composite scores is similarly strong ($r(203) = .89$, $p < .0001$). There is some evidence that these two composite scores are beginning to "decouple" slightly in the older group ($r = .64$ in the 8- to 15-year-old group versus $r = .77$ in the 3- to 6-year-old group), but this difference was not significant (*Fisher's z*, $p = .07$).

Other Demographic Differences

When adjusted for age, there were no significant "effects" of gender, mother's education, or family income on the total group's Toolbox

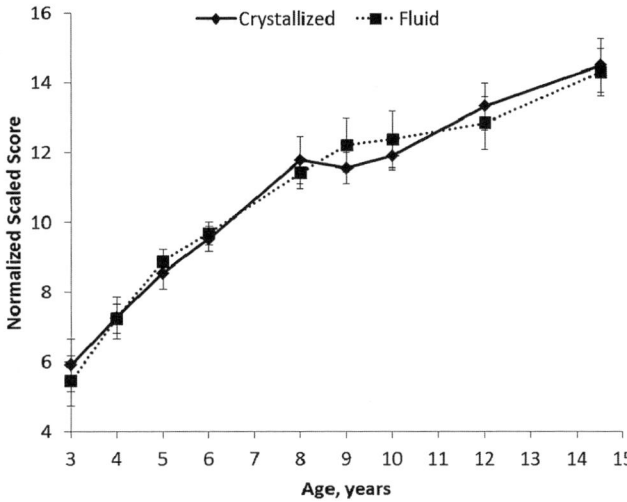

FIGURE 13.—Performance on the Toolbox Crystallized Cognition Composite and the Toolbox Fluid Cognition Composite across age groups. Error bars represent ±2 SE.

Crystallized Cognition Composite, Toolbox Fluid Cognition Composite, or Toolbox Total Composite. There were statistically significant ethnicity effects, albeit with small effect sizes (ESs = .25, .28, .29), on the age-adjusted Toolbox Crystallized Cognition Composite ($F(2, 192) = 4.96$, $p = .008$), Fluid Cognition Composite ($F(2, 194) = 5.93$, $p = .003$), and Total Composite ($F(2, 194) = 7.80$, $p = .0006$). On each of the composite scores, Caucasian children scored higher than African American children.

Relations With Health Status and School Performance

Again using the total participant sample (ages 3–15), children's reported health status was significantly related (but with small effect sizes) to the age-adjusted Toolbox Crystallized Cognition Composite ($F(1, 199) = 7.62, p = .006$; $ES = .21$), Fluid Cognition Composite ($F(1, 199) = 4.03$, $p = .046$; $ES = .15$) and Total Composite ($F(1, 199) = 8.41$, $p = .004$; $ES = .20$). In each case the children described as having "excellent" health performed somewhat better than those described as having less than excellent (poor to very good) health.

Associations of Toolbox composite scores with reported school performance were assessed only in the older (school age, 8–15) children, because many of the younger children were not yet in formal school settings. In the older children, school performance was strongly associated (medium to large effect sizes) with age-adjusted scores on the Toolbox Crystallized Cognition Composite ($F(1, 77) = 34.48$, $p < .0001$; $ES = .86$), Fluid Cognition Composite ($F(1, 77) = 13.48$, $p = .0004$; $ES = .65$), and Total Composite ($F(1,

77) = 34.72, $p < .0001$; $ES = .85$). Children who were reported to have "above average" school performance (vs. average or below average) scored consistently higher on all composite scores. Similarly, children who were reported to have needed "special" (remedial) classes or tutoring in school performed worse on age-adjusted Toolbox Crystallized ($F(1, 75) = 10.53$, $p = .002$; $ES = .67$), Fluid ($F(1, 75) = 3.25$, $p = .075$; $ES = .44$), and Total ($F(1, 75) = 12.03$, $p = .0009$; $ES = .72$) composite scores.

Construct Validity

Convergent

As noted above, comparisons of results on the NIH Toolbox and validation composite scores required separate analyses for the two age groups (3–6 and 8–15 years) because established measures were different at different ages (see also Chapter 1). In Table 21 are correlations between analogous Toolbox and validation composite scores for the two age groups. These results show excellent convergent validity for the full and short composite scores in both age groups: median correlations of .88 for Crystallized, .70 for Fluid, and .88 for Total.

Discriminant

Only modest evidence for discriminant validity is provided by slightly lower correlations between Toolbox Crystallized and Validation Fluid Composite scores (median $r = .71$) and between Toolbox Fluid and Validation Crystallized Composite scores ($r = .72$). These latter results should be considered in light of the very high correlation between the Toolbox Crystallized and Fluid Composite scores themselves ($r = .89$ for the full sample).

Evidence of discriminant validity for the short battery composites (for children with ages of 3–6 years only) consisted of somewhat lower correlations for nonanalogous than those for analogous composites: the correlation between

TABLE 21

PEARSON CORRELATIONS BETWEEN FULL AND SHORT NIH TOOLBOX CB AND VALIDATION COMPOSITE SCORES FOR YOUNGER (3–6 YEARS) AND OLDER (8–15 YEARS) CHILDREN (ALL $ps < .0001$; dfs IN PARENTHESES)

	Full Composites		Short Composites
	Age 3–6	Age 8–15	Age 3–6
Crystallized	.88 (114)	.90 (85)	.73 (109)
Fluid	.78 (111)	.70 (85)	.69 (111)
Total	.90 (114)	.88 (85)	.80 (113)

© 2006–2012 National Institutes of Health and Northwestern University.

Short Toolbox Crystallized and Validation Fluid Short Composite scores was .48 ($df = 107$, $p < .0001$), and that between Short Toolbox Fluid and Validation Crystallized Short Composite scores was .67 ($df = 112$, $p < .0001$).

Developmental Trajectories of Toolbox Versus Validation Composites

Given the results in Table 21, it should not be surprising that the Toolbox and Validation composite scores show very similar developmental trajectories (age effects) in childhood (see Figure 14a and b). Although there appears to be a sharp increase in the slope in Figure 14b after the age of 10, this probably is an artifact based upon the need to include more than one age in the last two categories (because of small sample sizes). Also similar to results for the Toolbox measures presented above, there were no significant gender effects on age-adjusted validation composite scores for either age group. Maternal education was related to validation composite scores only in the 3- to 6-year-old group (all $ps < .05$). Also only in the younger group, family income was associated with just one validation composite (Crystallized; $p < .05$).

As noted above, significant ethnicity effects were seen on all Toolbox composite scores when the full age range (3–15 years) was considered, reflecting somewhat better cognitive performance in the Caucasian than in the African American children. However, when the smaller age subgroups were analyzed separately, most of these differences became nonsignificant trends (exceptions were Toolbox Fluid and Total Composite scores in the 3–6 year olds). Similarly, in these age subgroups the ethnicity group differences in the validation composite scores showed mostly nonsignificant trends (exceptions were Validation Fluid Composite scores in the 3–6 year olds, and Validation Crystallized Composite scores in the 8–15 year olds).

As was reported above in relation to the Toolbox composite scores, strong and consistent relations were found between all validation composite scores and reported school functioning in the older, school-age group. This was true in relation to parental reports of children's overall school performance (above average vs. below average or average) as well as reports about the needs for special classes or tutoring.

DISCUSSION

The results from the validation study suggest that the proposed Toolbox Crystallized Cognition, Fluid Cognition, and Cognitive Function (i.e., total) Composite scores provided reliable measures of important aspects of cognition for children between the ages of 3 and 15. Although the subgroup of our participants that was reassessed in this study was relatively small ($n = 66$), the test–retest reliability estimates on the Toolbox composite scores ($rs = .92-.96$) are comparable to those seen with well-established cognitive

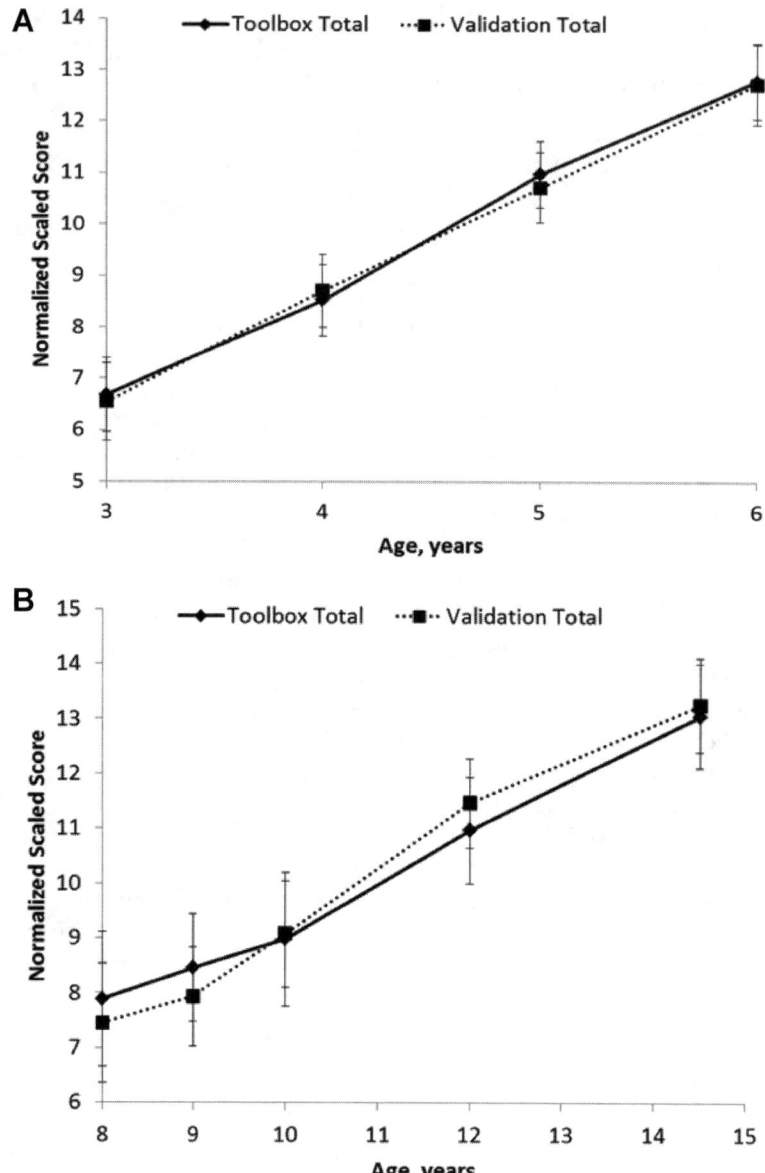

FIGURE 14.—Performance on the Toolbox Cognitive Function Composite (Total) and the Validation Total Composite across ages, plotted separately for younger (3–6 years) and older (8–15 years) children. Error bars represent ±2 *SE*.

summary scores in the literature (e.g., IQ scores on the Wechsler intelligence scales; Sattler, 2001; WAIS-III WMS-III Technical Manual, 1997).

The longitudinal data in this study also indicate a modest practice effect for the Toolbox Fluid Cognition Composite but not the Toolbox Crystallized Cognition Composite. This is expected, because of the types of abilities that are reflected in these composite scores. Tests of "fluid" cognition involve new learning and adapting to novel stimuli and task requirements; when such tests are repeated the examinee tends to show improved performance because the test stimuli and required tasks are more familiar (less novel). This benefit of prior test exposure is not as likely when previously learned knowledge and skills (crystallized cognition) are being assessed. Other examples of this fluid versus crystallized difference include repeated administrations of intelligence test batteries, where Perceptual Organization and Processing Speed (fluid) composite scores show more improvement than "crystallized" measures of Verbal Comprehension (WAIS-III WMS-III Technical Manual, 1997). On the other hand, even the largest practice effect observed for a Toolbox composite was rather modest (average of only about ½ scaled score point on the Toolbox Fluid Cognition Composite, with a medium effect size of .54). Nevertheless, longitudinal studies that use NIH Toolbox Fluid Cognition Composite or any other fluid cognition measures must control for practice effects to avoid misinterpreting these as "real" improvements due to development or some form of intervention (medical or educational).

Associations with age were based on the data from the full sample of children ($N = 208$). Across the age span represented in this sample (3–15 years), all three CB composite scores demonstrated a strong, linear developmental trajectory. Two points about this are worth noting. First, whereas in adults fluid and crystallized abilities tend to diverge with older age because of greater "normal aging" effects on fluid cognition (e.g., Heaton et al., 2003), during childhood the developmental effects on the two types of cognition show parallel positive trends (Sattler, 2001). Indeed, in Figure 13, the mean age trajectories of the Toolbox Crystallized and Fluid Cognition Composite scores are virtually overlapping. Furthermore, to our knowledge the CB is unique in its ability to track with the same instruments both developmental effects and effects of adult aging across the entire lifespan (ages 3–85 years).

In this chapter we also examined possible relations between multiple demographic factors and children's performance on the CB. By far, children's age was the most powerful demographic predictor. Once age was corrected, there were no significant effects of gender, or SES as indexed by mother's education level or family income. Consistent with typical findings in adult groups (Heaton et al., 2003, 2004; Heaton, Ryan & Grant, 2009; Norman et al., 2011), Caucasian children performed somewhat better than their African American counterparts on the Toolbox composite scores. The effect sizes of these differences were "small," however, and lower than is typically seen in studies of adult cognition. Nevertheless, when normative standards are being used to evaluate possible developmental or acquired cognitive *disorders*, failure to adjust for even small demographic effects can increase classification errors (e.g., Heaton et al., 2003).

Although the current study focused on a rather restricted (12-year) age range in childhood, we were unable to find comparable validation tests that allowed us to explore convergent and discriminant validity across these ages. For this reason, CB versus validation associations and comparisons had to be done separately for the 3–6 year olds and the 8–15 year olds. The analyses provided evidence for excellent convergent validity in both age groups. There was less support for discriminant validity when comparing Toolbox Fluid and Crystallized Cognition Composite scores with Validation Crystallized and Fluid Composite scores, respectively. This is not surprising, given the exceptionally strong, positive age effects on all cognitive measures in this study (both Toolbox and validation), as well as robust correlations between the Toolbox Fluid and Crystallized Cognition Composite scores across the full childhood age span (3–15 years).

There may be situations where researchers choose to use the single Toolbox Cognitive Function Composite as a measure of overall cognitive ability in children. Although there were strong correlations between the Toolbox Fluid and Crystallized Cognition Composite scores, it is unlikely that this collection of neuropsychological tests is simply measuring one underlying ability or cognitive factor (see Mungas et al., Chapter 7, this volume). There continues to be much debate about the nature and development of fluid and crystallized abilities and general intelligence (see Blair, 2006). Research on newer measures of children's fluid cognition is needed, particularly examining how they relate to the development of crystallized abilities and the underlying brain maturation associated with the development of these skills. The CB is currently being utilized in a large NIH-funded multi-site study of brain development, and appears to hold promise in this regard.

Our assessments of children's health status and academic performance were limited to rather gross indicators by maternal reports. The health status ratings, in particular, lacked specificity, and their small (but statistically significant) effects on the age-corrected CB composite scores probably were due to particular health problems that may have influenced cognitive development and/or educational experiences in some children. Future research should be directed at validating the CB measures for detecting effects on cognition of specific health conditions of interest (e.g., trauma or infections involving the brain, developmental disorders, other chronically disabling conditions).

Perhaps this study's most impressive evidence of the CB Composite scores' criterion validity (other than the convergent validation with established measures) was their strong associations with maternal ratings of children's school performance and needs for special classes or tutoring (large effect sizes). This might not be surprising for the Toolbox Crystallized Cognition Composite, because this composite reflects previously acquired semantic knowledge (vocabulary) and reading skills that are both products of more or less successful educational experiences. Although the Toolbox Fluid Cognition Composite does not directly reflect what the child has learned in the past, it does indicate the status of other cognitive abilities that may be considered necessary to succeed in future schoolwork (i.e., attention, working memory, processing speed, episodic memory, and executive function). These findings suggest, therefore, that the CB composite scores may have validity for assessing aspects of children's cognition that are important for educational success.

In our experience, it is sometimes more difficult to administer the entire CB to children under age 7 years than to school age children. Younger children may require more time to become familiar with the task instructions and may fatigue more easily, despite the relatively short time required to administer the CB. Examination of potential "short form" scores for children ages 3–6 years was promising. The use of scores from two CB tests to create the Short Toolbox Fluid Cognitive score produced results that were very similar to the Toolbox Fluid Composite score (which includes scores from five tests). However, reliability of the Vocabulary measure (as a single measure of crystallized ability) was much lower than expected in the youngest children. This will be reassessed during norming. The computer response format used with the validation sample was a touch screen and it was noted that some of the youngest children had difficulty with the touch screen. In the norming version the touch screen has been replaced with two button keys (arrow keys) which will likely reduce unintended response errors. The national norming study will involve a larger, more representative sample of both children and adults, and is expected to provide further confirmation of the reliability and validity of the Crystallized, Fluid, and Total Composite scores introduced here.

REFERENCES

Benedict, R. (1997). *Brief visuospatial memory test-revised*. Odessa, FL: Psychological Assessment Resources.
Blair, C. (2006). How similar are fluid cognition and general intelligence? A developmental neuroscience perspective on fluid cognition as an aspect of human cognitive ability. *Behavioral and Brain Sciences,* **29**, (2), 109–125 (with Commentary, 125–160).
Cattell, R. B. (1971). *Abilities: Their structure, growth, and action*. Boston: Houghton Mifflin.
Delis, D. C., Kramer, J. H., & Kaplan, E. (2001). *The Delis–Kaplan executive function system*. San Antonio, TX: The Psychological Corporation.

Dunn, L. M., & Dunn, D. M. (2007). *Peabody picture vocabulary test* (4th ed.). San Antonio, TX: Pearson.

Gronwall, D. M. (1977). Paced auditory serial-addition task: A measure of recovery from concussion. *Perceptual and Motor Skills*, **44**, 367–373.

Heaton, R. K., Miller, S. W., Taylor, J. T., & Grant, I. (2004). *Revised comprehensive norms for an expanded Halstead–Reitan Battery: Demographically adjusted neuropsychological norms for African American and Caucasian adults*. Lutz, FL: Psychological Assessment Resources, Inc.

Heaton, R. K., Ryan, L., & Grant, I. (2009). Demographic influences and use of demographically corrected norms in neuropsychological assessment. In I. Grant & K. M. Adams (Eds.), *Neuropsychological assessment of neuropsychiatric and neuromedical disorders* (pp. 127–155). New York: Oxford University Press.

Heaton, R. K., Taylor, M. J., & Manly, J. (2003). Demographic effects and use of demographically corrected norms with the WAIS-III and WMS-III. In D. S. Tulsky, D. H. Saklofske, G. J. Chelune, R. K. Heaton, R. J. Ivnik, R. Bornstein, et al. (Eds.), *Clinical interpretation of the WAIS-III and WMS-III* (pp. 181–210). San Diego, CA: Academic Press.

Horn, J. L. (1968). Organization of abilities and the development of intelligence. *Psychological Review*, **75**, 242–259.

Horn, J. L. (1970). Organization of data on life-span development of human abilities. In L. R. Goulet & P. B. Baltes (Eds.), *Life-span developmental psychology: Research and theory* (pp. 423–466). New York: Academic Press.

Horn, J. L., & Cattell, R. B. (1967). Age differences in fluid and crystallized intelligence. *Acta Psychologica*, **26**, 107–129.

Korkman, M., Kirk, U., & Kemp, S. (2007). *NEPSY-II* (2nd ed.). San Antonio, TX: Harcourt Assessment.

Li, S.-C., Lindenberger, U., Hommel, B., Aschersleben, G., Prinz, W., & Baltes, P. (2004). Transformations in the couplings among intellectual abilities and constituent cognitive processes across the life span. *Psychological Science*, **15**, 155–163.

Norman, M. A., Moore, D. J., Taylor, M., Franklin, D., Cysique, L., Ake, C., et al. (2011). Demographically corrected norms for African Americans and Caucasians on the Hopkins Verbal Learning Test-Revised, Brief Visuospatial Memory Test-Revised, Stroop Color and Word Test, and Wisconsin Card Sorting Test 64-Card Version. *Journal of Clinical and Experimental Neuropsychology*, **4**, 1–11. EPub May 2011.

Rey, A. (1964). *L'examen clinique en psychologie*. Paris: Presses Universitaires de France.

Sattler, J. M. (2001). *Assessment of children: Cognitive applications*. San Diego, CA: Jerome M. Sattler, Publisher.

The Psychological Corporation. (1997). *WAIS-III WMS-III technical manual*. San Antonio, TX: The Psychological Corporation.

Wechsler, D. (2002). *Wechsler preschool and primary scale of intelligence-3rd edition (WPPSI-III)*. San Antonio, TX: The Psychological Corporation.

Wechsler, D. (2003). *Wechsler intelligence scale for children* (4th ed.). San Antonio, TX: The Psychological Corporation.

Weintraub, S., Dikman, S. S., Heaton, R. K., Tulsky, D. S., Zelazo, P. D., Bauer, P. J., et al. (2013). Cognition Assessment using the NIH Toolbox. *Neurology*, **80**, S54–S64.

Wilkinson, G. S., & Robertson, G. J. (2006). *Wide range achievement test 4 professional manual*. Lutz, FL: Psychological Assessment Resources.

IX. NIH TOOLBOX COGNITION BATTERY (CB): SUMMARY, CONCLUSIONS, AND IMPLICATIONS FOR COGNITIVE DEVELOPMENT

Patricia J. Bauer and Philip David Zelazo

ABSTRACT This monograph describes the creation of the National Institutes of Health Toolbox Cognition Battery (NIH Toolbox CB) and reports validation data for children ages 3–15 years. Individual chapters described measures of executive function, episodic memory, language, working memory, speed of processing, and attention. Separate chapters were devoted to the factor structure of the test battery and composite measures of cognitive health (Total Composite, Fluid Composite, Crystallized Composite). In all cases, the NIH Toolbox CB measures showed sensitivity to age-related changes across the 3- to 15-year range as well as test/retest reliability. The measures also demonstrated adequate to excellent convergent validity, and there was evidence of greater discriminant validity among older than younger children. Confirmatory factor analyses revealed five- and three-factor models for the older (8–15 year olds) and younger (3–6 year olds) children, respectively. The correlation between the Fluid and Crystallized Composite scores was higher among the younger than the older children. The overall pattern is suggestive of greater differentiation of cognitive abilities with age. The strong psychometric properties of the CB and its apparent sensitivity to patterns of developmental change suggest that it is an important advance in the study of cognitive development and has the potential to substantially accelerate discoveries through use of common methods across disparate laboratories and even disciplines.

The National Institutes of Health Toolbox Cognition Battery (NIH Toolbox CB) is an initiative of the Neuroscience Blueprint, designed to accelerate discoveries and reduce the burden of nervous system disorders, in part by providing a common set of assessment tools that can be used across

---

Corresponding author: Patricia J. Bauer, Department of Psychology, 36 Eagle Row, Emory University, Atlanta, GA 30322, email: patricia.bauer@emory.edu

laboratories, populations, and disciplines to measure cognitive, emotional, sensory, and motor health across the lifespan, from ages 3–85 years. The NIH Toolbox CB is unique in its continuity across childhood and adolescence, early adulthood, and old age, and distinguished in its brevity and its suitability for repeated administration in longitudinal designs. It also is freely available to researchers for use, making it an ideal vehicle for creation of a common currency among disparate studies.

Individual chapters in this monograph described the process by which particular cognitive subdomains were selected, the rationale for test design, and data on the psychometric properties of the tests during childhood (ages 3–15 years), including sensitivity to age-related differences, test/retest reliability, and construct validity. Finally, separate chapters were devoted to discussion of the factor structure of the test battery, with emphasis on differences between younger and older children, and the development of composite measures of cognitive health derived from the individual assessments. In this final chapter, we present brief summaries of the rationale for development of the CB and the major findings from the validation study, followed by discussion of the implications of the CB for the study of cognitive development, the limitations of the battery, and directions for further development of the instrument.

MOTIVATION AND RATIONALE FOR DEVELOPMENT OF THE NIH TOOLBOX CB

Selection of Domains and Subdomains

As described in Chapter 1, one of the first steps in construction of the CB was selection of the subdomains of cognition to be assessed. This step was necessary because of the mandate that the CB be relatively brief, such that the entire battery could be administered in 20 min for children (30 min for adults). This necessitated selection of some subdomains at the exclusion of others. The selection of subdomains was based on: (1) their importance to the course of development and aging; (2) their significance for health and success in education and, in adults, for work; (3) their validation with respect to known underlying brain mechanisms; and (4) their ease of measurement and translation into brief test instruments. With these criteria in mind, under the guidance of a Steering Committee, teams of experts and potential "end users" were polled and interviewed to determine their priorities for assessment. The information was supported by thorough reviews of the literature on cognitive function and development. These steps resulted in selection of the subdomains represented in the CB, namely, executive function (including both cognitive flexibility and inhibitory control), episodic memory, language (including both vocabulary comprehension and reading decoding), working memory, and processing speed; the measures to assess these subdomains are described in Chapters 2–6, respectively. Assessment of the factor structure of these subdomains was discussed in Chapter 7. In addition, as described in Chapter 8, scores from the measures were combined to create composite scores that address the perceived need for global measures of cognitive function.

The developers are keenly aware that the selection of some subdomains and not others has implications for the scope of assessment that the CB provides. For example, 43% of initial respondents ranked visuospatial functions as one of the four most important subdomains to assess. Yet because the subdomain ranked below several others, and given the constraints on the duration of the CB, the decision was made not to include a measure of visuospatial function. As a result, visuospatial function, and its potential implications for overall cognitive health, cannot be assessed. A related, yet different, concern is that the need to keep the instrument brief means that even the subdomains included in the CB are not assessed in depth. Researchers whose primary interest is in one of the subdomains may want to use instruments that provide more intensive and extensive assessments of that particular subdomain. Finally, the CB is not intended as a neuropsychological examination instrument. Researchers whose primary interest is in assessment of neuropsychological status are advised to use instruments that have been shown to be sensitive to neurological insult or injury; the neuropsychological sensitivity of the CB has yet to be assessed. These caveats aside, the NIH Toolbox CB shows substantial promise as a brief assessment of cognitive function (as discussed below).

Selection of Measures

As described in Chapter 1, the measures of each subdomain to be included in the CB needed to be brief, easy to administer, available free of charge, and suitable for use across the entire age range of 3–85 years. To satisfy these criteria, new measure were developed. Some measures were modeled after tests available in the literature whereas others were based on experimental work. In some cases, measures were modeled after those in the adult literature and were scaled down to be appropriate for children (e.g., the measure of processing speed). In other cases (e.g., executive function and episodic memory), measures were modeled after those in the developmental literature and were scaled up to be appropriate for adults. All measures underwent pilot testing prior to test for validation.

VALIDATION: SUMMARY OF MAJOR FINDINGS

To determine the reliability and construct validity of the instruments as measures of the target subdomains, the Cognition Team conducted a validation study across the 3- to 85-year age range. Resulting data were used to test the sensitivity of the measures to age-related change, the test/retest reliability of the measures, and to test the construct validity of the measures. We also examined the factor structure of the CB and used the data to construct composite scores reflective of overall cognitive heath, and both fluid and crystallized abilities. We also examined relations between the composite scores and several demographic variables. The findings are summarized below.

Sensitivity to Age-Related Change

In all cases, the CB measures showed sensitivity to age-related changes across the 3- to 15-year age range. Table 22 includes a summary of the correlations with age across all measures. As is apparent in the table, correlations ranged from .77 (processing speed: Toolbox Pattern Comparison Processing Speed Test) to .86 (reading: Toolbox Oral Reading Recognition Test).

Test/Retest Reliability

In all cases, across the 3- to 15-year age range, the CB measures showed high correlations between the first and the second administration and thus demonstrated test/retest reliability. Table 22 includes a summary of the

TABLE 22

Summary of Correlations of NIH Toolbox CB Measures With Age and of Estimates of Test/Retest Reliability

	Ages 3–15 Years	
Domain/Measure	Correlation With Age	Test/Retest Reliability
Executive function		
Toolbox Flanker Inhibitory Control and Attention Test	.83	.91
Toolbox Dimensional Change Card Sort (DCCS) Test	.84	.92
Episodic memory		
Toolbox Picture Sequence Memory Test	.78	.76
Language		
Toolbox Picture Vocabulary Test	.81	.81
Toolbox Oral Reading Recognition Test	.86	.97
Working memory		
Toolbox List Sorting Working Memory Test	.77	.86
Processing speed (5 year olds youngest age tested)		
Toolbox Pattern Comparison Processing Speed Test	.77	.84
Toolbox Processing Speed Composite	.77	.84

© 2006–2012 National Institutes of Health and Northwestern University.

correlations between first and second administration. As is apparent in the table, correlations ranged from .76 (episodic memory: Toolbox Picture Sequence Memory Test) to .97 (reading: Toolbox Oral Reading Recognition Test). Correlations in this range are considered evidence of excellent test–retest reliability.

Construct Validity

Assessment of the validity of the CB measures of the subdomains was complicated by a number of factors. For many subdomains, there was no single measure that could be used across the 3- to 15-year age range (which was, of course, one of the motivations for development of new measures). Indeed, in one case (processing speed), there was no measure that was appropriate for use to test convergent validity for 3 and 4 year olds; for this reason, the youngest children tested for the convergent validity of the NIH Toolbox Pattern Comparison Processing Speed Test were 5 year olds. In addition, selection of the most appropriate measures of discriminant validity was difficult because especially for the youngest children (a) there are relatively few tests of specific cognitive functions; and (b) the established measures available (e.g., the PPVT-IV) frequently are used as proxies of general intelligence, which obviously would be expected to overlap with function in any specific domain. The outcome of the tests for construct validity must be evaluated with these constraints in mind.

Convergent Validity

In Table 23, we summarize the results of tests of convergent validity for executive function, episodic memory, working memory, and processing speed. In each of these subdomains, different measures were used for the younger and older children in the sample. As is apparent from Table 23, the correlations were all statistically significant. In most cases, the correlations were moderate in magnitude. Higher correlations with the established measures were observed for the measures of vocabulary and reading. For both of these subdomains, the same validation measures were used for the younger and older children. Across the 3- to 15-year age range, the CB measure of vocabulary, the TPVT, was correlated .90 with the PPVT-IV. The CB measure of reading, the TORRT was correlated .96 with the WRAT and .87 with the PPVT-IV.

Discriminant Validity

In Table 24, we summarize the results of tests of discriminant validity for executive function, episodic memory, working memory, and processing speed. Although in most cases, the same discriminant measures were used for the younger and older children, the results are provided separately for the younger and older children in order to permit evaluation of the relative

TABLE 23
SUMMARY OF CORRELATIONS BETWEEN NIH TOOLBOX CB MEASURES AND MEASURES OF CONVERGENT VALIDITY

Domain/NIH Toolbox CB Measure	Validation Measure	Age Group	
		3–6 Years	8–15 Years
Executive function			
Toolbox Flanker Inhibitory Control and Attention Test	WPPSI-III Block Design	.63	
	D-KEFS Inhibition		.36
Toolbox Dimensional Change Card Sort (DCCS) Test	WPPSI-III Block Design	.68	
	D-KEFS Inhibition		.61
Episodic memory			
Toolbox Picture Sequence Memory Test	NEPSY-II Sentence Repetition	.50	
	RAVLT/BVMT-R composite		.47
Working memory			
Toolbox List Sorting Working Memory Test	NEPSY-II Sentence Completion	.57	
	Letter/Number Sequencing		.57
Processing speed (5 year olds youngest age tested)			
Toolbox Pattern Comparison Processing Speed Test	WPPSI-III/WISC-IV Processing Speed Composite	.43	.40
	PASAT		.39
Toolbox Processing Speed Composite	WPPSI-III/WISC-IV Processing Speed Composite	.37	.44
	PASAT		.34

Note. PPVT-IV, Peabody Picture Vocabulary Test-4th Edition; WRAT-R, Wide Range Reading Test-Revised; WPPSI-III, Wechsler Preschool and Primary Intelligence Test, 3rd Edition; WISC-IV: Wechsler Intelligence Scale for Children, 4th Edition; NEPSY-II, Developmental Neuropsychological Assessment, 2nd Edition; PASAT, Paced Auditory Serial Attention Test; D-KEFS, Delis–Kaplan Executive Function Scales.© 2006–2012 National Institutes of Health and Northwestern University.

TABLE 24

Summary of Correlations Between NIH Toolbox CB Measures and Measures of Discriminant Validity

Domain/NIH Toolbox CB Measure	Validation Measure	Age Group	
		3–6 Years	8–15 Years
Executive function			
Toolbox Flanker Inhibitory Control and Attention Test	PPVT-IV	.72	.45
Toolbox Dimensional Change Card Sort (DCCS) Test	PPVT-IV	.79	.54
Episodic memory			
Toolbox Picture Sequence Memory Test	PPVT-IV	.58	.28
Working memory			
Toolbox List Sorting Working Memory Test	PPVT-IV	.63	.45
	WCST-64		.42
	D-KEFS		.45
Processing Speed (5 year olds youngest age tested)			
Toolbox Pattern Comparison Processing Speed Test	PPVT-IV	.44	.36
Toolbox Processing Speed Composite	WAIS-IV Letter-Number Sequencing		.20 ns
	PPVT-IV	.60	.52
	WAIS-IV Letter-Number Sequencing		.42

Note
PPVT-IV, Peabody Picture Vocabulary Test-4th Edition; WRAT-R, Wide Range Reading Test-Revised; WPPSI-III, Wechsler Preschool and Primary Intelligence Test, 3rd Edition; WCST-64, Wisconsin Card Sorting Test-64 Card version; D-KEFS, Delis–Kaplan Executive Function Scales; WAIS-IV: Wechsler Adult Scale of Intelligence, 4th Edition.

strength of the correlations for the measures of convergent and discriminant validity. As is apparent from Table 23, for the subdomains of executive function, episodic memory, working memory, and speed of processing, the correlations not only were statistically significant, but typically were of moderate magnitude. In addition, in each case, the correlations were higher for the younger children than for the older children. The significance of this pattern was discussed in detail in Chapter 7. The pattern is consistent with the suggestion of differentiation of cognitive domains over the course of development. The one exception to the pattern was the Toolbox Pattern Comparison Processing Speed Test measure of processing speed. For the older children, the WAIS-IV Letter-Number Sequencing test was not significantly correlated with the Toolbox Pattern Comparison Processing Speed Test. The CB measures of vocabulary (TPVT) and reading (TORRT) both were correlated .53 with the measures of discriminant validity (RAVLT/BVMT-R in both cases).

Relative Strengths of Correlations

In evaluation of the validity of the assessments as measures of the target constructs, the most important question is whether correlations with the measures of convergent validity were higher than those of discriminant validity. For the younger children, in the subdomains of executive function, episodic memory, and working memory, convergent validity correlations were not greater than discriminant validity correlations. In contrast, for the subdomains of processing speed, vocabulary, and reading, the expected pattern obtained: indices of convergent validity were nominally higher than indices of discriminant validity. For the older children, the expected pattern was more readily apparent. That is, indices of convergent validity were nominally higher than indices of discriminant validity. Thus, overall, but especially for children ages 8–15 years, the CB measures demonstrated construct validity.

As discussed in Chapter 7, as well as in the next section, this overall pattern is consistent with existing evidence that neurocognitive functions undergo differentiation with development. Although this means that measures of some functions necessarily lack discriminant validity at younger ages, they are nonetheless reliable and developmentally sensitive at these ages. The limitation on discriminant validity early in development is tolerable, given the importance of having consistent measures of these functions as they become differentiated from general cognitive skills.

Factor Structure of the NIH Toolbox CB

The CB was designed to measure six subdomains of cognitive function: executive function, episodic memory, language, working memory, processing speed, and sustained attention, and as discussed in Chapter 7, factor analysis of the validation data from adults (reported elsewhere) supported a six-factor solution. As summarized in Chapter 7, we used the results of the validation study reported in this monograph to test whether the assessment battery also revealed six factors in participants ages 3–15 years. As reported in Chapter 7, we found that, in the 3- to 15-year age range, the assumption of a six-dimensional structure was not well supported by the data. The fit between the assumption and the data was better for the older children (8–15 year olds), where the data supported a five-factor solution, than for the younger children (3–6 year olds), where only three factors emerged.

For the 8- to 15-year-old children and adolescents, the five factors identified in the confirmatory factor analysis of the dimensional structure of the CB and the validation tests were Working Memory, Episodic Memory,

Vocabulary, Reading, and a combined Executive Function/Processing Speed factor. For the 3- to 6-year-old children, the three factors found were Vocabulary; Reading; and Fluid Abilities, which included the CB measures of executive function, episodic memory, working memory, and processing speed. Moreover, there was higher intercorrelations among factors among the younger children compared with the older children, and among the older children compared with adults. For both the older and younger groups of children, age was strongly correlated with the latent variables, likely reflecting the profound influences of brain development coupled with life experiences on cognitive abilities.

The results of the analysis of the factor structure of the CB are consistent with suggestions in the existing literature of increasing differentiation of cognitive abilities with development. The pattern is predicted based on consideration of neurocognitive development, which in general involves the increasing functional specialization of neural systems (e.g., Johnson & Munakata, 2005). The pattern also has been born out empirically. For example, within the subdomain of executive function, whereas a three-factor model provides an excellent fit to data from adults (e.g., Miyake et al., 2000), data from preschool-age children are more consistent with a one-factor model (e.g., Wiebe, Espy, & Charak, 2008; Wiebe et al., 2011). These patterns make all the more remarkable the finding that in both the younger and older age groups, Vocabulary and Reading—both measures of language skills and abilities—were clearly separable factors. That is, for both age groups, model fit was higher when Vocabulary and Reading were treated as separate factors as opposed to a common factor of language.

Composite Scores From the NIH Toolbox CB and Relations With Demographic Variables

Composite Scores

One of the findings of the early surveys and interviews with experts and potential "end users" of the CB (described briefly earlier in this chapter and in detail in Chapter 1) was the perceived need for a single measure of cognitive development. The factor analysis of the CB, just described, supports the suggestions that already by age 3 years, and increasingly with development, cognitive function may best be characterized in terms of multiple factors, each of which may be expected to have its own course of development. Nevertheless, a single composite measure of overall cognitive function is often desirable—for example in large epidemiological or population studies in which assessment of cognition is not the major focus. Accordingly, the Cognition Team used the data from the validation study to develop a single composite measure. We also developed measures of both components of the two-component theory of intellectual development (Cattell, 1971;

Horn, 1968, 1970), namely, fluid and crystallized abilities. Fluid abilities are those that require new learning and adaptive problem solving, and crystallized abilities are more dependent on past learning experiences. The process and results are described in detail in Chapter 8, and summarized only briefly here.

The general composite score and both of the component scores (fluid and crystallized abilities) were highly sensitive to age-related developmental change. Across the 3- to 15-year age span, correlations with age were .88 for the Total Composite, .86 for the Fluid Composite, and .87 for the Crystallized Composite. An interesting trend in the data was that the correlation between the Fluid and Crystallized Composite scores was higher among the younger children (3–6 year olds) than among the older children (8- to 15-year-old): correlations of .77 and .64, respectively. Consistent with the findings from the factor structure analysis discussed above, this pattern is suggestive of greater differentiation of cognitive abilities with age. As might be expected, the composite scores also demonstrated excellent test/retest reliability, and excellent convergent validity in both the younger and older age groups of children. Only modest evidence for divergent validity was obtained, however.

Relations With Other Demographic Variables

As discussed in Chapter 8, when scores were age adjusted, there were no significant relations between child gender, mother's education, or family income and the Total Composite, Fluid Composite, or Crystallized Composite. There were statistically significant ethnicity effects, reflecting higher scores for Caucasian children than African American children. However, the effect sizes associated with ethnic differences were small for all three composites. Moreover, when the younger and older age subgroups were analyzed separately, most of the differences became nonsignificant trends. Within the sample as a whole, all three composites were associated with better health, as measured by parent report, albeit with small effect sizes. Finally, within the older age group only, children who were reported to have "above average" school performance scored consistently higher on all three composites, whereas children who were reported to have needed "special" (remedial) classes or tutoring in school scored consistently lower. Relations with school performance were not evaluated for the younger age group since many had not yet begun formal schooling. As a whole, these findings provide evidence of the ecological validity of the CB.

IMPLICATIONS FOR THE STUDY OF COGNITIVE DEVELOPMENT

One of the most obvious implications of the CB for the study of cognitive development is that it provides a tool that can be used across the life span. The cognitive development literature is populated by tasks and measures that are useful for one age period or another, but which have limited utility over large tracts of developmental time. In contrast, the CB can be used from ages 3 to 85 years. This feature of the battery has implications for both cross-sectional and longitudinal designs. In cross-sectional studies, use of measures that are equally appropriate for younger and older participants will reduce concerns about potential floor and ceiling effects for younger and older participants, respectively. In longitudinal studies, the same task can be used at earlier and later assessment points, which will simplify data analysis and allow greater confidence in interpretation. The possibility of significant practice effects was examined for each of the measures individually and also for the composite scores (Chapter 8). The Crystallized Composite evidenced virtually no practice effect. However, the fact that both the Total Composite and the Fluid Composite scores showed significant effects must be taken into consideration in interpretation of longitudinal studies using the CB. The concern may be lessened somewhat by the observation that the magnitude of practice effect was not significantly correlated with age for any of the composites.

Development of the CB also facilitates analysis of the process of differentiation of cognitive domains with development. The fact that six subdomains of cognition can be measured relatively quickly and efficiently makes it possible to examine the course of development of each subdomain over time, as well as whether, and if so, how, relations among them may change with age. The chapters on the factor structure (Chapter 7) and the derivation of composite scores (Chapter 8) from the CB both revealed evidence of differentiation of cognitive domains with age. With the exception of vocabulary and reading, which were differentiated even among the youngest children (3–6 years), older children (8–15 years), showed greater evidence of differentiation than did younger children. Yet even among the older children, and in contrast to adults (see Chapter 7), the subdomains of executive function and processing speed remained relatively undifferentiated. Also, with development, fluid and crystallized abilities became more differentiated. These findings are consistent with suggestions that neurocognitive development in general involves greater functional specialization of both neural systems (e.g., Johnson & Munakata, 2005) and cognitive functions (e.g., Wiebe et al., 2008, 2011). The CB is a new tool in the research arsenal that will permit further test and evaluation of these interesting hypotheses.

LIMITATIONS OF THE NIH TOOLBOX CB

The CB is an important advance in the study of cognitive development and has the potential to substantially accelerate discoveries through use of common methods across disparate laboratories and even disciplines. It thus can be expected to reduce the burden of nervous system disorders. The battery also has some limitations, however. Ironically, perhaps the most salient limitation simultaneously is a source of great strength of the instrument, namely, that it is brief. Because it is brief, the CB permits assessment of key aspects of cognitive health in studies in which time is limited—for example, with child participants, or in studies that seek to examine relations between cognition and other domains of function. In cases where a more intensive assessment of cognition (or a particular subdomain) is required, it is possible to supplement the CB with more comprehensive assessments of targeted cognitive subdomains. Coupling the broad-based CB with more in-depth measures will permit researchers to evaluate the target domain against the backdrop of overall cognitive health.

A second limitation of the CB already has been addressed in this chapter, namely, the fact that not all subdomains of cognition are included in the battery. Although not all subdomains are included, the CB features assessments of those domains that the majority of experts and potential "end users" identified as the most important to measure. Thus, although the instrument is not exhaustive of all aspects of cognition, it does provide a state-of-the-art window onto critical features of cognitive health. The most obvious way to address this limitation is to supplement the CB with assessments of domains not currently sampled by it (e.g., visuospatial functions).

A third limitation of the CB is that it is not currently designed for use with children younger than 3 years of age. For researchers who work with infants and toddlers, the reasons for the lower-bound on the instrument are relatively obvious: children much younger than the age of 3 years cannot be expected to make reliable (or any) verbal responses or to comprehend verbal instructions. Moreover, infants and very young children have limited fine-motor control and thus could not be expected to meet demands to move cursors or click mouse buttons. Some measures (e.g., the Toolbox DCCS Test and the Toolbox Flanker Inhibitory Control and Attention Test) are currently being modified for use with younger children for possible inclusion in the National Children's Study. For now, however, the limitation remains: the CB is not useful for infants and children younger than 3 years of age. This fact limits the utility of the instrument for cross-sectional and longitudinal studies designed to cross the boundary of 3 years. In some cases, it may be possible to adapt the current CB assessments for use with infants and children under the age of 3. However, as the Cognition Team found when constructing instruments for children ages 3 and older, in some cases it likely will be more feasible to adapt infant measures for use with older children than to attempt the adaptation in the other direction.

FURTHER DEVELOPMENT OF THE NIH TOOLBOX CB

The NIH Toolbox CB has come a very long way in a relatively short period of time (development of the instrument began in 2006). Yet significant additional steps remain to be taken. We discuss three of the most obvious here. First, the CB will undergo testing with a larger number of children, adolescents, and adults, to establish norms for performance. The target sample for norming is 4,000 children, adolescents, and adults ages 3–85 years. The sample will be representative of the population of the United States, in terms of race and ethnicity, gender, and socioeconomic status, among other variables. A subset of those assessed will be retested 1 week and 3 months later, to determine the test/retest reliability of the battery, its sensitivity to age-related change over short periods of time (in children and elderly adults, in particular), and its susceptibility to practice effects.

The second direction for further development is to validate and norm a Spanish-language version of the instrument. Spanish is spoken as the primary language by an estimated 16% of the population in the United States and by many countries in the developed and developing world. These facts made it critical that a Spanish-language version of the CB be developed. The need for a Spanish-language version was recognized at the outset of development of the CB and suitability for translation was one of the features considered throughout development of the instrument. The norming study just described will be conducted simultaneously in English and Spanish, and will be the major avenue for validation and further adjustment (in the domains of Vocabulary and Reading in particular) of the Spanish version of the CB.

A third direction for further development is to test the CB with populations of children and adults suffering from neurological insult or injury or neurocognitive developmental disorders. The validation study included participants with a broad range of backgrounds and ability levels. Yet it was not designed specifically to evaluate cognitive health in children with special needs or neurocognitive disabilities. The goal of use of the CB as a common assessment tool across laboratories, populations, and disciplines will be facilitated by further development of the instrument for use with even more diverse populations.

CONCLUSION

The NIH Toolbox CB provides measures of six important cognitive subdomains across the lifespan. In this monograph, we presented data on the performance of the battery in the 3- to 15-year age range. The measures are sensitive to age-related changes between 3 and 15 years and each of the individual assessments demonstrates high levels of test/retest reliability. The measures also are correlated with established measures of the target constructs, indicating adequate to excellent convergent validity. Evidence of discriminant validity is not as strong, especially among the 3- to 6-year-old children. Rather than as a limitation of the measures, however, we may view this as an indication of the gradual differentiation of cognitive subdomains over the course of child development. The latter interpretation is consistent with analyses of the factor structure of the battery, and with the patterns of correlation between composite measures of cognitive function derived from the individual assessment tools. Importantly, performance on the CB is related to overall health and to school performance, suggesting it has ecological validity as well. Important next steps in development of the CB are to establish norms of performance for diverse populations, across the entire age span of 3–85 years, for both English and Spanish speakers. With this step, the CB will be well situated for use across laboratories, populations, and disciplines to measure cognitive function across the lifespan, from ages 3 to 85 years. The CB is further distinguished in its brevity and its suitability for repeated administration in longitudinal designs. It has been available to researchers free of charge since October 2012 (see www.nihtoolbox.org for current information), making it an ideal means of establishing commonality across data sets from disparate studies, thus further accelerating the pace of progress in diagnosis and treatment of mental disorders.

REFERENCES

Cattell, R. B. (1971). *Abilities: Their structure, growth, and action.* Cambridge, UK: Cambridge University Press.

Horn, J. L. (1968). Organization of abilities and the development of intelligence. *Psychological Review,* **75,** 242–259.

Horn, J. L. (1970). Organization of data on life-span development of human abilities. In L. R. Goulet & P. B. Baltes (Eds.), *Life-span developmental psychology: Research and theory* (pp. 423–466). Waltham, MA: Academic Press.

Johnson, M. H., & Munakata, Y. (2005). Processes of change in brain and cognitive development. *Trends in Cognitive Science,* **9**(3), 152–158.

Miyake, A., Friedman, N. P., Emerson, M. J., Witzki, A. H., Howerter, A., & Wager, T. D. (2000). The unity and diversity of executive functions and their contributions to complex "frontal lobe" tasks: A latent variable analysis. *Cognitive Psychology,* **41,** 49–100.

Wiebe, S. A., Espy, K. A., & Charak, D. (2008). Using confirmatory factor analysis to understand executive control in preschool children: I. Latent structure. *Developmental Psychology,* **44,** 575–587.

Wiebe, S. A., Sheffield, T., Nelson, J. M., Clark, C. A. C., Chevalier, N., & Espy, K. (2011). The structure of executive function in 3-year-olds. *Journal of Experimental Child Psychology,* **108,** 436–452.

APPENDIX A

Significance values of pairwise comparisons (least squares means) between age groups (years) for each of the NIH toolbox cognition battery (CB) measures, based on normalized, scaled scores.

Toolbox Dimensional Change Card Sort Test

	3	4	5	6	8	9	10	11–13	14–15
3		.0094	<.0001	<.0001	<.0001	<.0001	<.0001	<.0001	<.0001
4	.0094		<.0001	<.0001	<.0001	<.0001	<.0001	<.0001	<.0001
5	<.0001	<.0001		0.2853	.0003	<.0001	<.0001	<.0001	<.0001
6	<.0001	<.0001	.2853		.0033	.0003	<.0001	<.0001	<.0001
8	<.0001	<.0001	.0003	.0033		.5759	.4095	.0246	<.0001
9	<.0001	<.0001	<.0001	.0003	.5759		.7933	.0855	<.0001
10	<.0001	<.0001	<.0001	<.0001	.4095	.7933		.1376	<.0001
11–13	<.0001	<.0001	<.0001	<.0001	.0246	.0855	.1376		.0027
14–15	<.0001	<.0001	<.0001	<.0001	<.0001	<.0001	<.0001	.0027	

Toolbox Flanker Inhibitory Control and Attention Test

	3	4	5	6	8	9	10	11–13	14–15
3		.0010	<.0001	<.0001	<.0001	<.0001	<.0001	<.0001	<.0001
4	.0010		<.0001	<.0001	<.0001	<.0001	<.0001	<.0001	<.0001
5	<.0001	<.0001		.0356	<.0001	<.0001	<.0001	<.0001	<.0001
6	<.0001	<.0001	.0356		<.0001	<.0001	<.0001	<.0001	<.0001
8	<.0001	<.0001	<.0001	<.0001		.9825	.8017	.0774	<.0001
9	<.0001	<.0001	<.0001	<.0001	.9825		.7848	.0810	<.0001
10	<.0001	<.0001	<.0001	<.0001	.8017	.7848		.0441	<.0001
11–13	<.0001	<.0001	<.0001	<.0001	.0774	.0810	.0441		.0123
14–15	<.0001	<.0001	<.0001	<.0001	<.0001	<.0001	<.0001	.0123	

Corresponding author: Philip David Zelazo, Institute of Child Development, University of Minnesota, 51 East River Road, Minneapolis, MN 55455-0345, email: zelazo@umn.edu

Toolbox Picture Sequence Memory Test

	3	4	5	6	8	9	10	11–13	14–15
3		.0053	<.0001	<.0001	<.0001	<.0001	<.0001	<.0001	<.0001
4	.0053		.0053	<.0001	<.0001	<.0001	<.0001	<.0001	<.0001
5	<.0001	.0053		.0008	<.0001	<.0001	<.0001	<.0001	<.0001
6	<.0001	<.0001	.0008		.0023	<.0001	<.0001	<.0001	<.0001
8	<.0001	<.0001	<.0001	.0023		.0831	.0043	.0253	.0010
9	<.0001	<.0001	<.0001	<.0001	.0831		.2531	.5908	.1265
10	<.0001	<.0001	<.0001	<.0001	.0043	.2531		.5558	.7319
11–13	<.0001	<.0001	<.0001	<.0001	.0253	.5908	.5558		.3432
14–15	<.0001	<.0001	<.0001	<.0001	.0010	.1265	.7319	.3432	

Toolbox Picture Vocabulary Test

	3	4	5	6	8	9	10	11–13	14–15
3		.0033	<.0001	<.0001	<.0001	<.0001	<.0001	<.0001	<.0001
4	.0033		.0595	.0061	<.0001	<.0001	<.0001	<.0001	<.0001
5	<.0001	.0595		.4587	<.0001	<.0001	<.0001	<.0001	<.0001
6	<.0001	.0061	.4587		<.0001	<.0001	<.0001	<.0001	<.0001
8	<.0001	<.0001	<.0001	<.0001		.6982	.5090	.0436	<.0001
9	<.0001	<.0001	<.0001	<.0001	.6982		.2951	.0167	<.0001
10	<.0001	<.0001	<.0001	<.0001	.5090	.2951		.1692	.0001
11–13	<.0001	<.0001	<.0001	<.0001	.0436	.0167	.1692		.0154
14–15	<.0001	<.0001	<.0001	<.0001	<.0001	<.0001	.0001	.0154	

Toolbox Oral Reading Recognition Test

	3	4	5	6	8	9	10	11–13	14–15
3		.0214	<.0001	<.0001	<.0001	<.0001	<.0001	<.0001	<.0001
4	.0214		<.0001	<.0001	<.0001	<.0001	<.0001	<.0001	<.0001
5	<.0001	<.0001		<.0001	<.0001	<.0001	<.0001	<.0001	<.0001
6	<.0001	<.0001	<.0001		<.0001	<.0001	<.0001	<.0001	<.0001
8	<.0001	<.0001	<.0001	<.0001		.7445	.9304	.0007	<.0001
9	<.0001	<.0001	<.0001	<.0001	.7445		.6831	.0002	<.0001
10	<.0001	<.0001	<.0001	<.0001	.9304	.6831		.0011	<.0001
11–13	<.0001	<.0001	<.0001	<.0001	.0007	.0002	.0011		.0293
14–15	<.0001	<.0001	<.0001	<.0001	<.0001	<.0001	<.0001	.0293	

Toolbox List Sorting Working Memory

	3	4	5	6	8	9	10	11–13	14–15
3		.0052	.0001	<.0001	<.0001	<.0001	<.0001	<.0001	<.0001
4	.0052		.1806	.0002	<.0001	<.0001	<.0001	<.0001	<.0001
5	.0001	.1806		.0211	<.0001	<.0001	<.0001	<.0001	<.0001
6	<.0001	.0002	.0211		<.0001	<.0001	<.0001	<.0001	<.0001
8	<.0001	<.0001	<.0001	<.0001		.1408	.2828	.0510	.0010
9	<.0001	<.0001	<.0001	<.0001	.1408		.6881	.6126	.0750
10	<.0001	<.0001	<.0001	<.0001	.2828	.6881		.3676	.0281
11–13	<.0001	<.0001	<.0001	<.0001	.0510	.6126	.3676		.2210
14–15	<.0001	<.0001	<.0001	<.0001	.0010	.0750	.0281	.2210	

Toolbox Pattern Comparison Processing Speed Test

	3	4	5	6	8	9	10	11–13	14–15
3		.0017	<.0001	<.0001	<.0001	<.0001	<.0001	<.0001	<.0001
4	.0017		.0001	<.0001	<.0001	<.0001	<.0001	<.0001	<.0001
5	<.0001	.0001		.1241	.0002	<.0001	<.0001	<.0001	<.0001
6	<.0001	<.0001	.1241		.0093	<.0001	<.0001	<.0001	<.0001
8	<.0001	<.0001	.0002	.0093		.1639	.0085	.0122	<.0001
9	<.0001	<.0001	<.0001	<.0001	.1639		.2080	.2488	.0012
10	<.0001	<.0001	<.0001	<.0001	.0085	.2080		.9304	.0504
11–13	<.0001	<.0001	<.0001	<.0001	.0122	.2488	.9304		.0441
14–15	<.0001	<.0001	<.0001	<.0001	<.0001	.0012	.0504	.0441	

COMMENTARY

COMMENTARY ON *ZELAZO AND BAUER (EDITORS), NATIONAL INSTITUTES OF HEALTH TOOLBOX COGNITION BATTERY (CB): VALIDATION FOR CHILDREN BETWEEN 3 AND 15 YEARS*

Nathan A. Fox

In April of 2006, Richard Gershon, who is the Principal Investigator of the contract from NIH for the development of the NIH Toolbox, contacted me and asked me to join the executive committee of the project. The committee was comprised of himself, David Cella (a health psychologist and currently Chair of the Department of Medical Health at Northwestern University Medical School), Richard J. Havlik (a physician and epidemiologist working for WESTAT), and Hugh Hendrie (who was a Professor of Geriatric Medicine at Indiana University). The NIH representative on the committee was Molly Wagster, who is affiliated with the National Institute on Aging. My responsibilities included representing the needs of the pediatric population (children between the ages of 3 and 17 years) for this large and complex project.

The NIH Toolbox contract stated that the instruments to be developed and selected for inclusion should assess individuals beginning at age 3 years and through age 85 years. The tasks were to have reasonable test–retest reliability as well as adequate convergent and divergent validity. Other requirements stipulated in the contract included a time constraint for the administration of the entire toolbox, the need for measures to be in the public domain (meaning no intellectual property issues since the NIH Toolbox is to be posted on the web for public use) and importantly, that the measures have links to the emerging neuroscience research literature so that they could tap known circuitry in the brain. Four broad domains were identified in the contract for the identification and development of assessment tools:

Corresponding author: Nathan A. Fox, Department of Human Development and Quantitative Methodology, University of Maryland, College Park, MD 20742, email: fox@umd.edu

cognition, socio-emotional health, motor, and sensory processes. Each of these domains was chaired by an individual expert in the field, though not necessarily someone with expertise in development. For example, the chair of the Cognition Domain Team was Professor Sandra Weintraub from Northwestern University whose area of expertise is attention in aging and dementia, and the chair of the Socio-emotional Health Domain Team was Paul Pilkonis from the University of Pittsburgh who studies personality and emotions in adults. The need for input from developmental psychologists was evident and so the task was to identify people who were willing to become involved in the project who could provide consultation and in important instances provide instruments that they had developed. In the case of the cognition domain, these individuals included Phil Zelazo (University of Minnesota) Patricia Bauer (Emory University), Kathy Hirsh-Pasek (Temple University), Roberta Gollinkof (University of Delaware), and Jean Berko Gleason (Boston University). In addition to these individuals, Mike Posner, Joel Kaplan, and Adele Diamond were consulted with regard to measures of attention and executive function.

As described in the paper by Weintraub et al. (Chapter 1, this volume), a number of subdomains were identified for each of the four major domains. In the case of Cognition, the subdomains of executive function and sustained attention, working memory, processing speed, attention shifting, language, reading, and episodic memory were identified. Although the original contract requirements stated that the NIH Toolbox should cover the age range from 3 to 85 years, inclusion of tasks that covered each of these subdomains for children as young as 3 years of age was far from a certainty when he started. First, it was not clear if tasks could be identified that would meet the test criteria of the toolbox (test–retest reliability, convergent and discriminant validity). Given the variability in young children's performance on experimental tasks assessing cognitive skills, identifying or developing tasks that met statistical criteria might not be possible. Second, there was some debate in the executive committee as to whether it was possible or even necessary to assess similar constructs across the broad age range. Some members argued that certain constructs were not present in early childhood, emerging only later in childhood. And third (and perhaps most important at the time) funds for what was called "the pediatric option" were not a certainty, given the funding level on the contract and the cost required for a large undertaking necessary to create measures for children ages 3–17 years. In order to confirm funding for the Pediatric measures a meeting was convened with the heads of all of the NIH institutes to hear presentations by Richard Gershon and myself on the importance of this initiative. After this meeting, the funds for the pediatric option were approved. Subsequent to this meeting a Pediatric Working Group was organized that would have oversight on the development of instruments for children across all domains. Among the issues addressed by the Working Group were the establishment of a set of principles that would be applicable across domains for the assessment of children. These principles included the importance of having an examiner present, the need for clear instructions, the importance of practice trials to insure that children understand the tasks, the importance of feedback after practice trials and during task performance, the importance of engaging the child and motivating performance, and monitoring the pace of assessment. One of the big issues here was building in flexibility for breaks and pauses in administration of different tasks. The software programmers had to modify their code to allow examiners to include these breaks so as to provide flexibility in administration. In addition to these issues the working group dealt with ergonomic issues that arose having to do with the equipment being used for testing, the type of furniture used, and the importance of the testing environment to elicit best performance. For example, in the current monograph a number of the assessment instruments utilized a touch screen during the validation phase of test development. Subsequent examination of the data and report from those who administered the tasks found that there were both technical and methodological problems with the touch screens. The screens were often too sensitive or not sensitive enough to touch, and the position of the child's hands prior to the onset of a trial had to be monitored. In some instances this led to inaccurate assessment of reaction times. Subsequent to the validation phrase, a decision was reached to change to a mouse rather than use the touch screen as it was found that even 3 year olds were able to control the buttons on a mouse with a high degree of success.

A number of instruments were identified for each subdomain in cognition and multiple discussions and reviews were undertaken to compare the merits of each. In addition, a number of instruments were identified that had been used by researchers in laboratory studies at various ages within the age span of interest. These included the Dimensional Change Card Sort, developed by Phil Zelazo and used widely in cognitive development research, and the Imitation Based Assessment of Memory developed by Patricia Bauer and used to study the development of episodic memory. In addition, the NIH Toolbox appropriated for the assessment of attention the Flanker task developed by Jin Fan and Michael Posner, and adapted existing tasks for assessing processing speed, vocabulary, reading, and working memory. There was a detailed and elaborate process between identification of the tasks and their administration in the validation phase. Stimuli had to be selected, decisions regarding presentation (voice instructions vs. administrator live instruction) had to be made, and pilot testing for ease and efficacy of administration of the tasks had to be completed. Subsequently, a pre-validation study was conducted in which measures were assessed for convergent and divergent validity. With promising findings, the next phase of development was initiated, the validation study of these measures.

In the validation phase over 200 children between the ages of 3–15 years were recruited and were assessed on the final battery of cognitive tasks. In addition, composite scores as well as the factor structure of the tasks were examined. The current monograph presents the results of this effort and as well, provides the reader for each of the individual tasks, a brief window into the decisions for the choice and development of each instrument. In addition, each paper provides the reader with a rationale for the inclusion of a particular subdomain and the link between performance on that subdomain, in relation to the current literature in cognition and development as well as links to neural function. Both these explications provide the interested reader and potential user of the instruments with a grounding in the constructs thought to underlie the subdomain under study as well as its underlying neural circuitry. Both behavior and brain links provide a foundation for choice of the subdomain and its utility in future studies. For example, Tulsky et al. (Chapter 5, this volume) provide an in-depth discussion of the construct of working memory, its relation to other memory processes, as well as suggestions about the neural circuitry or network that is thought to underlie working memory ability. Finally, two papers, Mungas et al. (Chapter 7, this volume) and Akshoomoff et al. (Chapter 8, this volume) present the reader with information on the factor structure and composite scores (respectively) of the tasks, their convergent and discriminant validity.

The findings presented across the papers in this monograph are remarkably consistent across measures demonstrating good test–retest reliability for individual tasks, and adequate convergent and divergent validity. In some instances, identifying a "gold standard" for a particular subdomain and age was challenging. For example, as a measure of sustained attention, parents of 3–4 year olds were asked to complete the short form of the Children's Behavior Questionnaire, which provided a subscale called Attention Focusing that was used to compare children's attention scores derived from the Flanker. Nevertheless, across tasks and measures the data for both the 3–6 year olds and the 8–15 year olds are respectable.

There are a number of interesting and important findings in this group of papers. One involves the correlation between the variables from each task and age. For some tasks, the correlations with age were high and positive indicating a linear relation between performance and age (e.g., pattern comparison; Carlozzi et al., Chapter 6, this volume). For others, the correlation with age for the 3–6 year olds was positive and high but much lower for the 8- to 15-year-old group (e.g., the Picture Sequence Memory Test where the correlation between performance and age was .69 for the 3–6 year olds and .26 for the 8- to 15-year-old; see Bauer et al., Chapter 3, this volume). Similar disparities between the two sets of correlations are evident for list sorting and the measures of attention (inhibition, sustained attention, and set shifting; see Zelazo et al., Chapter 2, this volume). Why might that be? Examination of the figures (e.g., Figure 3 for the Toolbox DCCS Test, the Flanker inhibitory control measure, and the Flanker attention measure, or Figure 2 for the Picture Sequence Memory Test, or Figure 2 for the List Sorting Working Memory Test) shows a relatively linear relation between age and test score through age 6, an asymptote or plateau around 9–10 years of age (for the List Sorting Working Memory Test) 10–14 years of age (for the Picture Sequence Memory Test) and a plateau for DCCS and Flanker measures (8–10 years of age). These deviations from linearity account for the lower correlations between task performance and age in these measures in the 8–15 year olds but more importantly, they suggest that skill development is not linear across age and that underlying changes (or lack thereof) in neural circuitry may underlie these nonlinearities. It would be interesting to examine in greater detail changes that occur in these skills post-adolescence where one might expect a second "growth spurt" in performance. One of the points of having developed tasks that can be administered across the age span is that hypothesized changes in performance as a function of age or brain growth can now be examined with a high degree of specificity. Indeed, examination of the composite scores (Figure 2a and b) displays just this plateau and renewed growth during adolescence. Figure 2A shows the linear increase in performance with age (between 3 and 6 years) while Figure 2b shows the plateau between 8 and 10 and then a linear increase from 10–14–15.

A second notable developmental finding described in this monograph can be found in the chapter by Mungas et al. (Chapter 7, this volume). This paper examined the factor structure of the tasks. There are interesting findings from the factor scores: at 3–6 years of age three factors emerge (reading, vocabulary, and the remaining measures which coalesce together). This changes in the 8–15 year olds with five factors now in evidence: vocabulary, reading, memory, working memory, and an executive function/processing speed factor. The differentiation from three to five factors speaks to the increasing specialization of skills with age and also links to what we know about increasing specialization of neural circuitry underlying these skills. The finding is particularly interesting given the discussion by Zelazo et al. (Chapter 2, this volume) regarding the diversity of executive function measures in adulthood and the findings of a single-factor solution in young children (Wiebe et al. 2008, 2011). As Zelazo et al. (Chapter 2, this volume) note, "it is possible … that EF becomes differentiated with age, although the use of different measures at different ages make this possibility difficult to assess." The value, then of the NIH Toolbox cognition measures is in the use of the *same* measure at different ages for each of the different EF skills with the result being a single factor encompassing all the EF skills. Interestingly, even in the 3–6 year olds, vocabulary and reading are their own factors suggesting that early in childhood, these skills are separate from EF skills.

A third notable finding from the paper by Akshoomoff et al. (Chapter 8, this volume) is with regard to the computation of composite scores reflecting crystallized and fluid intelligence. Fluid intelligence is thought to be less dependent upon learning experiences while crystallized abilities are more dependent upon experience and heavily influenced by education. The authors of this paper found first excellent test–retest correlations for both types of intelligence in ages 3–15 years. This was true also when two ages were examined separately (3–6 and 8–15 year olds). There was also a significant correlation between both types of intelligence with age although inspection of Figure 1 in the Akshoomoff et al. (Chapter 8, this volume) paper finds the same linear effect from ages 3–8 and 10 to 14–15 as reported above with a plateau between ages 8–10. Of interest is the strong correlation between fluid and crystallized intelligence. This is in contrast to the divergence of these two types of intelligence in adults (Heaton et al., 2003). It appears that through age 15 both types of intelligence follow similar trajectories of development and inter-connection. These results are somewhat at odds with the factor analytic results which find an increasing specialization with age in skill. It will be of interest to examine the pattern of these composite measures with a larger sample acquired during the norming phase of the project.

In sum, without too much bias, the development of the CB for the NIH Toolbox and the results contained in this monograph on the validation studies of this battery are a remarkable achievement. Each of the tasks displays solid psychometric properties. The factor structures of both young and older children confirm developmental expectations regarding the increasing specialization of skill and speak to findings from the neuroimaging literature that show increasing specificity of activation (as opposed to more global activation) during EF task performance. The tasks each presented here can be used by researchers as separate measures of the underlying constructs they are designed to represent. Alternatively, the tasks together can be summed to create composite scores reflecting both crystallized and fluid intelligence. The next phase, norming of these measures with a large and diverse population of children (both English and Spanish speaking) will provide the foundation for the use of the toolbox by the scientific community in the years to come.

CONTRIBUTORS

Marilyn Jager Adams (Ph.D., 1975, Brown University), is a Visiting Scholar in the Cognitive, Linguistic, and Psychological Sciences Department at Brown University. She is author of *Beginning to Read: Thinking and Learning about Print* (MIT Press). She chaired the Planning Committee and was a member of the Study Committee for the National Academy of Sciences' report, *Preventing Reading Difficulties in Young Children*. Since 1992 she has served on the Planning or Steering Committees for the *National Assessment of Educational Progress (NAEP)* in reading, and on the English/Language Arts Development Team for the *K-12 Common Core State Standards Initiative*.

Natacha Akshoomoff (Ph.D., 1992, San Diego State University/University of California, San Diego) is an Associate Professor in the Department of Psychiatry at the University of California, San Diego. Her research focuses on neuropsychological development of individuals with a variety of neurodevelopmental disorders, including autism, genetic conditions, and congenital brain injury. Her current research includes studies of typical development that bring together neuropsychological and academic assessment, neuroimaging, and genetics data.

Jacob E. Anderson (M.A., 2010, New Mexico State University) is a doctoral student in the Institute of Child Development at the University of Minnesota. He is actively involved in research examining the relations between brain development and the development of executive function, as well as how executive function can be promoted and improved in at-risk populations.

Patricia J. Bauer (Ph.D., 1985, Miami University) is Asa Griggs Candler Professor of Psychology, and Senior Associate Dean for Research, Emory College of Arts and Sciences, Emory University. She has received many awards, honors, and grants for her research on cognitive development. She serves on the Editorial Boards of *Developmental Review, Journal of Experimental Child Psychology*, and *Memory*. She is Editor of the *Monographs of the Society for Research in Child Development*, author of the award-winning volume, *Remembering the Times of Our Lives: Memory in Infancy and Beyond* (2007, Erlbaum), and

Co-Editor of the forthcoming *Wiley-Blackwell Handbook on the Development of Children's Memory*.

Jennifer L. Beaumont (M.S., 2002, University of North Carolina—Chapel Hill; Ph.D. Candidate, University of Illinois—Chicago) is a Statistical Analyst within the Department of Medical Social Sciences, at Northwestern University Feinberg School of Medicine. Her statistical interests include methodology to handle the unique issues of longitudinally assessed patient-reported outcomes.

David L. Blitz (Ph.D., 2012, Illinois institute of Technology) is a Senior Psychometrician at I/O Solutions, Inc. He has previously held positions at Motorola, Inc., Computer Adaptive Technologies, Inc., Promissor Inc., and the Department of Medical Social Sciences in the Northwestern University Feinberg School of Medicine. He also has served as an adjunct faculty member at the Chicago School of Professional Psychology and the Illinois Institute of Technology.

Beth G. Borosh (Ph.D., 2005, Nova Southeastern University) is an Assistant Professor in the Department of Psychiatry at Northwestern University Feinberg School of Medicine and Cognitive Neurology and Alzheimer's Disease Center. Her research focus is primarily in the areas of cognitive changes associated with normal aging and dementia, and the identification and assessment of neurocognitive constructs underlying health literacy in adults. She has been involved in several funded studies in these areas and clinical trials associated with the Cognitive Neurology and Alzheimer's Disease Center.

Noelle E. Carlozzi (Ph.D., 2005, University of Michigan) is an Assistant Professor in the Center for Rehabilitation Outcomes and Assessment Research within the Department of Physical Medicine and Rehabilitation, at the University of Michigan Medical School. Her research interests include neuropsychological assessment and the development of new outcomes measures (i.e., cognitive assessments and patient-reported outcomes). She is funded by the National Institute of Neurological Disorders and Stroke to develop and validate a new patient reported outcomes measure for use in individuals with Huntington disease.

Nicolas Chevalier (Ph.D., 2008, University of Provence, France) is a Research Associate at the Institute of Cognitive Science, University of Colorado Boulder. His research interests involve the development of executive function in children. In particular, he is interested in how children process environmental information to determine what goals they need to reach,

157

and ultimately how to behave adaptively. He examines the processes underlying goal representation in situations that require set-shifting or response inhibition, using behavioral, eye-tracking, and electrophysiological measures.

Sureyya S. Dikmen (Ph.D., 1973, University of Washington) is a Professor in the Department of Rehabilitation Medicine and Adjunct Professor in the Departments of Neurosurgery, and Psychiatry and Behavioral Sciences at the University of Washington. She has received awards and grants for her research on natural history of recovery in traumatic brain injuries (TBI) and clinical trials to improve outcomes. She has served on the editorial boards of the *Journal of the International Neuropsychological Society*, and the *Journal of Experimental and Clinical Neuropsychology*. She also has served on multiple TBI expert working groups, scientific advisory boards, and data and safety monitoring boards for the Centers for Disease Control and Prevention, NINDS, NIDRR, DoD, the Brain Injury Association of America, and the Institute of Medicine.

Kimberly A. Espy (Ph.D., 1994, University of Houston) is the Vice President for Research and Innovation, Dean of the Graduate School, at the University of Oregon. In addition to overseeing more than 70 graduate programs, Espy is responsible for more than 30 interdisciplinary research centers and institutes, ranging from the physical and life sciences to the social sciences and humanities disciplines. Espy, a trained clinical neuroscientist and professor of psychology, is the Director of the Developmental Cognitive Neuroscience Laboratory. In her federally funded research, she pioneered the integration of cognitive neuroscience tools and advanced multilevel growth modeling methods.

Nathan A. Fox (Ph.D., 1975, Harvard University) is Distinguished University Professor in the Department of Human Development at the University of Maryland. His research on infant temperament and the effects of early experience on brain and behavior is funded by the National Institutes of Health and he was recipient of a MERIT award from NICHD. He served as President of the International Society of Infant Studies and Division 7 of APA, is currently Associate Editor of the *International Journal of Behavioral Development*, and was Associate Editor for the journals *Psychophysiology* and *Developmental Psychology*, as well as Editor of *Infant Behavior and Development*. He is a Fellow of the Association for Psychological Science and the American Association for the Advancement of Science.

Richard C. Gershon (Ph.D., 1996, Northwestern University) is the Vice-Chairman for Research in the Department of Medical Social Sciences in the

Feinberg School of Medicine at Northwestern University. He serves as the principal investigator for the NIH Toolbox for the Assessment of Neurological and Behavioral Function and for the Patient Reported Outcomes Measurement Information Systems Technology Center. His research focuses on the development and application of computerized assessment tools across numerous disciplines.

Jean Berko Gleason (Ph.D., 1958, Harvard University) is Professor Emerita in the Department of Psychology at Boston University. A member of the Academy of Aphasia, she is past president of the International Association for the Study of Child Language and one of the founders of the field of psycholinguistics. She is the author and editor of leading textbooks in her field and many influential studies of language development in children and aphasia in adults. The eighth edition of her textbook *The Development of Language* has recently been published.

Roberta Michnick Golinkoff (Ph.D., 1973, Cornell University), is H. Rodney Sharp Professor of Education at the University of Delaware. She has held the John Simon Guggenheim Fellowship and the James McKeen Cattell prize, and she was named a Francis Alison Scholar, the highest honor given to faculty at the University of Delaware. She is the winner of the American Psychological Association's Distinguished Service to Psychological Science Award, and the Urie Bronfenbrenner Award for Lifetime Contribution to Developmental Psychology in the Service of Science and Society. Her research on language development, the benefits of play, and preschoolers' early spatial knowledge has resulted in numerous publications, including books for parents and practitioners. She is a co-founder of the Ultimate Block Party movement.

Richard J. Havlik (M.D., 1964, Northwestern University) retired from the National Institute on Aging (NIA), part of the National Institutes of Health, Bethesda, Maryland in 2005 and has been a medical consultant for Westat in Rockville, Maryland and ACRIA (AIDS Community Research Initiative of America) in New York City. From 1990 to his retirement, Dr. Havlik was Associate Director for Epidemiology, Demography, and Biometry and subsequently Chief of the Laboratory of Epidemiology, Demography, and Biometry in the Intramural Research Program at NIA. He directed a comprehensive program of research into the determinants and correlates of aging and age-associated diseases. His own research has covered a wide range of topics, including cardiovascular disease, cancer, cognitive functioning, dementia, and genetic epidemiology. Dr. Havlik has developed a current interest in the comorbidities associated with aging in HIV patients over 50 years of age.

Robert K. Heaton (Ph.D., 1972, University of Washington) is a Distinguished Professor and Vice Chair for Academic Affairs in the Department of Psychiatry, University of California at San Diego. He has authored or co-authored numerous scientific publications in neuropsychology and related fields, and has served on editorial boards of several scientific journals (*Journal of Consulting and Clinical Psychology, Journal of Clinical and Experimental Neuropsychology, Journal of the International Neuropsychological Society, The Clinical Neuropsychologist, Neuropsychology Review, PLoS-One*). He is a board certified neuropsychologist (ABPP-CN), is a Fellow of the American Psychological Association, the Association for Psychological Science and the National Academy of Neuropsychology, and is past president of the International Neuropsychological Society and the Clinical Neuropsychology Division of the American Psychological Association.

Kathryn Hirsh-Pasek (Ph.D., 1981, University of Pennsylvania) is the Stanley and Debra Lefkowitz Professor in the Department of Psychology at Temple University. She is the recipient of the American Psychological Association's Bronfenbrenner Award for Lifetime Contribution to Developmental Psychology in the Service of Science and Society, the American Psychological Association's Award for Distinguished Service to Psychological Science, the Great Teacher, and the Eberman Research Awards. Her research on early language development and infant cognition has been funded by the National Science Foundation and the National Institutes of Health and Human Development. She served as the Associate Editor of *Child Development* and as treasurer of the International Association for Infant Studies. Her book, *Einstein Never Used Flashcards: How Children Really Learn and Why They Need to Play More and Memorize Less* (Rodale Books), won the prestigious Books for Better Life Award as the best psychology book in 2003.

Robert V. Kail (Ph.D., 1975, University of Michigan) is a Distinguished Professor of Psychological Sciences at Purdue University. His research focuses on the development of processing speed during childhood and adolescence, as well as the impact of this change on other aspects of cognitive growth, such as growth in memory and reasoning. He served as Editor of *Psychological Science*, the flagship journal of the Association for Psychological Science, and currently is Editor of *Child Development Perspectives*.

Jennifer J. Manly (Ph.D., 1996, San Diego State University/University of California, San Diego) is an Associate Professor of Neuropsychology in Neurology at the G.H. Sergievsky Center and the Taub Institute for Research in Aging and Alzheimer's disease at Columbia University. Her research on cognitive and genetic aspects of aging and Alzheimer's disease among African Americans and Hispanics is funded by the National Institute on Aging and the

Alzheimer's Association. She is a Fellow of APA and serves on the US Department of Health and Human Services Advisory Council on Alzheimer's Research, Care and Services.

Dan Mungas (Ph.D., 1979, University of Montana) is a Professor of Neurology at the University of California at Davis. Dr. Mungas has been a leader in research on normal and abnormal cognitive aging in late life for many years, and has made important contributions to measurement of cognition in older populations with diverse linguistic and racial/ethnic backgrounds. Dr. Mungas has done groundbreaking work in applying item response theory methods to neuropsychological assessment, and leads an annual international conference on applications of modern psychometric methods to cognitive aging research.

Cindy J. Nowinski (Ph.D., 1991, Loyola University of Chicago; M.D., 2000, Northwestern University Feinberg School of Medicine) is a Research Assistant Professor and interim Director of Education within the Department of Medical Social Sciences, Northwestern University Feinberg School of Medicine. Her research interests include outcome measure development, evaluating the impact of chronic diseases and their treatments on patient-reported and clinical outcomes, and using health information technology to improve quality of care and patient outcomes.

Jennifer Richler (Ph.D., 2007, University of Michigan) is a Research Scientist in the Psychological and Brain Sciences department at Indiana University. She is funded by the Clinical and Translational Sciences Institute to conduct research on object exploration in children with autism spectrum disorders.

Deborah Schnipke (Ph.D., 1995, Johns Hopkins University) is a Psychometric Consultant, providing psychometric expertise for all aspects of testing programs in a variety of fields (e.g., certification and licensure testing, admissions testing, employment testing, and school assessment). She conducts psychometric analyses and evaluations of exams and testing programs, and introduces testing innovations. She has a substantial record of partnering with content specialists and software development teams to design, deploy, and maintain top-notch testing programs. She also has a strong research background, presenting results via publications, conferences, and training seminars.

Jerry Slotkin (Ph.D., 1990, University of Georgia) is a Senior Consulting Research Scientist with the Department of Medical Social Sciences at Northwestern University Feinberg School of Medicine. He has worked in leadership positions at a major assessment publisher and his career focus has been on the development of high-stakes assessments at the national, state, and local levels.

David S. Tulsky (Ph.D., 1989, University of Illinois—Chicago) is Professor and Director of Research in the Department of Physical Medicine and Rehabilitation and Director of the Center for Rehabilitation Outcomes and Assessment Research at the University of Michigan Medical School. He is nationally recognized as a leader in the area of patient-reported outcomes development and outcomes assessment. He has significant experience leading large-scale multicenter studies of rehabilitation outcomes, and is currently the principal investigator of several federally funded, multi-site projects related to the development of health-related quality of life instruments for rehabilitation populations.

Kathleen Wallner-Allen (Ph.D., 1996, University of Maryland, College Park) is a developmental psychologist and Senior Study Director at Westat. She has designed and implemented child assessments from infancy through early adolescence for national, large-scale longitudinal studies examining the role of home, early care and education, and school environments in children's cognitive, academic, social, and emotional development and health. Her research interests include executive function, attention, and academic achievement in typically developing children and children with learning disabilities.

Sandra Weintraub (Ph.D., 1978, Boston University) is Professor of Psychiatry, Neurology and Psychology at Northwestern University Feinberg School of Medicine in the Cognitive Neurology and Alzheimer's Disease Center. She has authored numerous articles and book chapters on the neuropsychology of dementia and aging, and on aphasia. She was one of two Scientific Honorees recognized at the Rita Hayworth Gala of the National Alzheimer's Association. She is the current president of the International Neuropsychological Society.

Keith Widaman (Ph.D., 1982, The Ohio State University) is a distinguished professor of psychology at the University of California at Davis. He conducts research on the development of children, adolescents, and young adults in the context of the family and broader behavioral and cultural contexts. Key in this research are longitudinal analyses that help identify effects of parents on their children and of children on their parents. In research on mental abilities, He studied the cognitive processes underlying numerical facility, especially as these processes change in nature and in speed of execution from childhood through early adulthood. He is a Fellow of the American Psychological Association, won the Cattell Award from the Society of

Multivariate Experimental Psychology, and is on the editorial boards of seven journals, including *Psychological Methods, Multivariate Behavioral Research, and Intelligence.*

Philip David Zelazo (Ph.D., 1993, Yale University) is the Nancy M. and John E. Lindahl Professor at the Institute of Child Development, University of Minnesota. His research has been recognized by numerous awards and honors, he serves on several editorial boards (e.g., *Child Development; Emotion; Development and Psychopathology*), and he is currently President of the Jean Piaget Society. In 2007, he was lead Editor of *The Cambridge Handbook of Consciousness*, and he is Editor of the 2013 two-volume *Oxford Handbook of Developmental Psychology.*

STATEMENT OF EDITORIAL POLICY

The SRCD *Monographs* series aims to publish major reports of developmental research that generates authoritative new findings and that foster a fresh perspective and/or integration of data/research on conceptually significant issues. Submissions may consist of individually or group-authored reports of findings from some single large-scale investigation or from a series of experiments centering on a particular question. Multiauthored sets of independent studies concerning the same underlying question also may be appropriate. A critical requirement in such instances is that the individual authors address common issues and that the contribution arising from the set as a whole be unique, substantial, and well integrated. Manuscripts reporting interdisciplinary or multidisciplinary research on significant developmental questions and those including evidence from diverse cultural, racial, and ethnic groups are of particular interest. Also of special interest are manuscripts that bridge basic and applied developmental science, and that reflect the international perspective of the Society. Because the aim of the *Monographs* series is to enhance cross-fertilization among disciplines or subfields as well as advance knowledge on specialized topics, the links between the specific issues under study and larger questions relating to developmental processes should emerge clearly and be apparent for both general readers and specialists on the topic. In short, irrespective of how it may be framed, work that contributes significant data and/or extends a developmental perspective will be considered.

Potential authors who may be unsure whether the manuscript they are planning wouldmake an appropriate submission to the SRCD *Monographs* are invited to draft an outline or prospectus of what they propose and send it to the incoming editor for review and comment.

Potential authors are not required to be members of the Society for Research in Child Development nor affiliated with the academic discipline of psychology to submit a manuscript for consideration by the *Monographs*. The significance of the work in extending developmental theory and in contributing new empirical information is the crucial consideration.

Submissions should contain a minimum of 80 manuscript pages (including tables and references). The upper boundary of 150–175 pages is more flexible, but authors should try to keep within this limit. If color artwork is submitted, and the authors believe color art is necessary to the presentation of their work, the submissions letter should indicate that one or more authors or their institutions are prepared to pay the substantial costs associated with color art reproduction. Please submit manuscripts electronically to the SRCD *Monographs* Online Submissions and Review Site (Scholar One) at http://mc.manuscriptcentral.com/mono. Please contact the *Monographs* office with any questions at monographs@srcd.org.

The corresponding author for any manuscript must, in the submission letter, warrant that all coauthors are in agreement with the content of the manuscript. The corresponding author also is responsible for informing all coauthors, in a timely manner, of manuscript submission, editorial decisions, reviews received, and any revisions recommended. Before publication, the corresponding author must warrant in the submissions letter that the study has been conducted according to the ethical guidelines of the Society for Research in Child Development.

A more detailed description of all editorial policies, evaluation processes, and format requirements can be found under the "Submission Guidelines" link at http://srcd.org/publications/monographs.

Monographs Editorial Office
e-mail: monographs@srcd.org

Editor, Patricia J. Bauer
Department of Psychology, Emory University
36 Eagle Row
Atlanta, GA 30322
e-mail: pjbauer@emory.edu

Note to NIH Grantees

Pursuant to NIH mandate, Society through Wiley-Blackwell will post the accepted version of Contributions authored by NIH grantholders to PubMed Central upon acceptance. This accepted version will be made publicly available 12 months after publication. For further information, see http://www.wiley.com/go/nihmandate.

SUBJECT INDEX

Page numbers in *italics* refer to tables and figures.

academic achievement, 17, 30, 121, 125–126
Accessibility Working Group, 8
age effects, 8–9, 103–118, 119–132, 136, *136*, 142, 143. *See also specific subdomain*
Alzheimer's disease, 5, 52
aphasiology, 53
attention, 16–17, 71. *See also* executive function
attention deficit hyperactivity disorder (ADHD), 4, 17, 72
auditory single word comprehension, 6
autism spectrum disorders, 4, 17, 72

brain
    anterior cingulat cortex, 73
    basal ganglia, 73
    cerebellum, 73
    cerebral hemisphere, 53
    cortex areas, 37, 104
    development, 104, 130, 141
    dorso-lateral prefrontal cortex, 73
    frontal cortex, 38
    frontal regions, 38
    fronto-parietal network, 72, 74
    gray matter, 105
    hippocampal region, 37
    limbic associational cortex, 37
    medial temporal cortex, 73
    medial-temporal lobe structures, 36, 38
    neocortex, 37
    occipital cortical areas, 105
    parietal cortex ventro cortex, 72–73
    parietal lobe, 73
    perisylvian area, 53
    polymodal prefrontal cortex, 37
    posterior cortex, 37

posterior regions, 73
prefrontal cortex (PFC), 6, 17, 20, 31, 37, 38, 73
primary sensory areas, 37
temporal lobe, 37
ventral prefrontal regions, 73
white matter, 90

cancer, childhood, 72
central executive, 71, 72
closed head injury, 90
Cognition Battery (CB)
    age-related change, 124, 136, *136. See also* age effects
    availability, 1
    demographic variables, 124–126, 141–142
    described, 1, 133–134
    composite scores, 119–132, 141–142, 143
    construct validity, 126–127, 137–140. *See also* construct validity
    convergent validity, 126, 137, *138*, 140. *See also* convergent validity
    correlations, strengths of, 140
    discriminant validity, 126–127, 130, 137, 139, *139*, 140. *See also* discriminant validity
    domain and subdomain selection, 134–135
    factor structure, 103–118, 140–141, 143
    further developments, 145
    general principles, 7
    implications for cognitive development, 142–143
    instrument selection, 7–9
    limitations, 143–144
    measurement selection, 2, 135
    motivation and rationale for development, 134–135
    populations and adaptability, 8
    Spanish versions, 7, 19, 49, 66, 117, 145, 146, 155
    test/retest reliability, 123–124, 136–137, *136*
    Toolbox Cognitive Function Composite, 120, 123–127, *128*, 142–143
    Toolbox Crystallized Cognition Composite, 120, 123–127, *125*, 129, 142–143
    Toolbox Dimensional Change Card Sort (DCCS) Test, 16, 19–20, 21–23, *21*, 26, 27, *27*, 28, *28*, 29–30, 92–93, 95, 96–98, *98*, *99*, 100, 113, 122, 144, *147*
    Toolbox Flanker Inhibitory Control and Attention Test, 16, 24–25, *24*, 26, 27, *27*, 28, *28*, 29–30, 93, 95, 96–98, *98*, *99*, 100, 122, 144, *147*
    Toolbox Fluid Cognition Composite, 120, 122, 123–127, *125*, 129, 142–143
    Toolbox List Sorting Working Memory Test, 70, 74–77, *75*, 78–79, *81*, 82–83, 113, 122, *149*
    Toolbox Oral Reading Recognition Test (TORRT), 49, 50, 53, 54, 57–59, *58*, 63–64, *64*, 65, 113, 114, *115*, 121, 137, 139, *148*

    Toolbox Pattern Comparison Processing Speed Test, 88, 91–93, *93*, 95–98, *98*, *99*, 100, 113, 122, 137, 139, *149*
    Toolbox Picture Sequence Memory Test (TPSMT), 34, 38–39, 42–43, *43*, 44–45, 113, 122, *148*
    Toolbox Picture Vocabulary Test (TPVT), 49, 53, 54–56, *55*, 61–63, *62*, *63*, 65, 113, 114, *115*, 121, 137, 139, *148*
    validation (major findings), 135–142
    working groups, 8
cognition, overall score, 119–132
cognitive control. *See* executive function (EF) and attention subdomain
composite scores, 119–121, 127–131, 135, 143
    age effects, 124, *125*
    analyses, 123
    construct validity, 126–127
    convergent validity, 126
    demographic differences, 124–125, 141–142
    discriminant validity, 126–127, 130
    method, 121–123
    NIH Toolbox CB measures, 121–122
    participants, 121
    relations with health status and school performance, 125–126
    results, 123–127
    test/retest reliability, 123–124
    trajectories of toolbox vs. validation composites, 127, *128*
    validation measures, 122–123, *126*
computer, 9, 21–22, 24, 40, 45, 65, 92, 98, 131, 144, 152
computerized adaptive testing (CAT), 46, 56, 65
Conduct Disorder, 4
confirmatory factor analysis (CFA)
    adults, 115, *115*
    age-related differences, 104–106, 115–117
    children 3–6 years of age, 110, *111*, 112, *112*
    children 8–15 years of age, *111*, 112–115, *114*
    construct validity, evaluating, 106
    data analysis, 108–110
    described, 103–104
    measures, 107, *107*
    method, 107–110
    participants, 107
    results, 110–115
construct validity, evaluating, 103–118, 126–127, 137–140. *See also specific subdomain*
convergent validity, 103, 106, 108–109, 113, 126, 137, *138*, 140. *See also specific subdomain*
crystallized capacities, 6, 35, 51, 115–116, 120, 121, 129–131, 136, 142–143, 154–155. *See also* semantic memory; vocabulary

Cultural Working Group, 8

declarative memory, 35
decoding automaticity, 52
developmental amnesia, 36, 38
developmental disability, 90
discriminant validity, 103, 106, 108–109, 120, 126–127, 130, 137, 139, *139*, 140. *See also specific subdomain*
dyslexia, 5, 72

education, maternal level, 121, 124, 127, 129, 142
encephalitis, 5
episodic buffer, 71
episodic memory subdomain, 2, 5, 34, 44–46, 134, 151
 age effects, 42–43, *43*, 44–45, 103, 115
 brain function relations, 37–38
 convergent validity measures, 41–42, 137, *138*, 140
 data analysis, 42
 defined, 34–35
 discriminant validity measure, 42, 45, 137, 139, *139*
 disease susceptibility, 5
 importance during childhood, 35–36
 measure development, 39–40, *39*
 method, 39–42
 participants, 39
 repeated testing, 43
 results, 42–44
 scoring, 40–41
 test/retest reliability, 43, 45
 toolbox measurement, 38–39
 validation measures, 41–42, 45
ethnicity. *See* race/ethnicity
executive attention, 19
executive function (EF) and attention subdomain, 2, 4–5, 29–33, 73–74, 134, 151
 age effects, 16, 27, *27*, *28*, 29–30, 103, 115, 143
 brain function relations, 105–106
 cognitive flexibility, 4, 5, 18, 19–20, 29
 components, 4–5, 6. *See also* working memory subdomain
 convergent validity measures, 25–26, 29, 137, *138*, 140
 data analysis, 26–27
 defined, 16–17
 discriminant validity measure, 26, 137, 139, *139*
 impairments, 4, 17
 importance during childhood, 17–18
 inhibitory control, 4, 5, 18, 19, 20–21, 29

method, 21–27
participants, 21
repeated testing, 28, 29
results, 27–29
structure, 18
test/retest reliability, 27, *28*
toolbox measurement, 19–21
validation measures, 5, 21–25, 25–26, 29, 116, 154
explicit memory. *See* declarative memory

family income. *See* socioeconomic status
fluid cognition, composite scores, 25, *107*, *109*, 110, *111*, 112, 115–116, 142–143, 154–155
focus of attention, 71

gender, 121, 124, 127, 129, 142, 145
Geriatric Working Group, 8

health, physical, 17, 121, 125–126, 130

language subdomain, 2, 5–6, 49, 134, 151
age effects, 61, *62*, 63, 103, 143
brain function relations, 53
components, 5–6
convergent validity, 61, 62–63, *63*, 64, 65, 137, *138*
data analysis, 61
defined, 50–51
discriminant validity, 61, 62–63, *63*, 64, 65, 140
disorders, 5, 52, 72
expressive, 53
importance during childhood, 51–52
method, 53–61
participants, 53–54
process indicators, 66
receptive, 53
repeated testing, 61–62, 63–64
results, 61–64
test/retest reliability, 61, 63, 65
validation measures, 54–59, 59–63, *63*, 64
leukemia, childhood acute lymphoblastic, 90
long-term memory, 35, 71

memory. *See* declarative memory; long-term memory; procedural memory; semantic memory; short-term memory; working memory
mouse (computer), 9, 45, 65, 144, 152
myelination, 37, 46, 90

SUBJECT INDEX

NIH Toolbox, 1–2, 7. *See also* Cognition Battery (CB)

oral reading, 6

pediatric option, 151
Pediatric Working Group, 8–9, 151
perceptual development, 30, 105
phenylketonuria, 90
phonological loop, 71, 83
prematurity, 72
procedural memory, 35
processing speed (PS) subdomain, 2, 6, 88, 134, 151
    age effects, 95, *96*, 98, *98*, 103, 115, 143
    biological substrates, 89–90
    cognitive processing, 89–90
    composite, 93, 96–97, *99*
    convergent validity, 94, 95, 96, *97*, 137, *138*
    data analysis, 94–95
    defined, 88–89
    discriminant validity, 94, 95, 96, *97*, 137, 139, *139*, 140
    importance during childhood, 89, 97
    in working memory, 70, 74
    measures, 92–93
    mental processing time, 6
    method, 92–95
    motor response time, 6
    neural impairments, 90
    participants, 92
    repeated testing, 96
    results, 95–97
    test/retest reliability, 95, 97, *98*
    validation measures, 90–92, 93–94, 97, 116, 137

race/ethnicity, 121, 127, 129, 142, 145
radiation treatment, 90
reaction time (RT), 88–89
reading decoding. *See* language subdomain

school achievement. *See* academic achievement
school readiness, 17
scores. *See* composite scores
semantic memory, 35, 51
set shifting, 19
short-term memory. *See* working memory subdomain
single word reading aloud, 6
socioeconomic status, 17, 30, 121, 124, 127, 129, 142, 145

stroke, 52, 53
substance dependence, 17
subdomain, 2, 3–6, *3*. *See also specific subdomain*

task switching, 19
temporolimbic epilepsy, 5
test/retest reliability, 123–124, 136–137, *136*. *See also specific domain*
touch-screen, 9, 21–22, 24, 40, 45, 65, 92, 98, 131, 152
traumatic brain injury, 72

validation measures, 2–3, 7, 10. *See also specific domain*
    by age group, 10, *12*
    CB measure, *11*
    composite measures, 122–123, *126*
    confirmatory factor analysis (CFA), 103–118
    pediatric validation sample, 9, *10*
    study, 9–10
visuospatial functions, 4
    as subdomain, 135, 144
    brain functions, 73–74
    episodic memory subdomain, 41
    language subdomain, 60
    memory, *11*
    sketchpad, 71, 73, 76, 82–83
vocabulary, 6, 45, 103, 131, 137, *138*, 143
    comprehension. *See* language subdomain
    receptive, 16, 20, 26, 30, 49, 50, 59, 79, 80, 82, 94, 95, 96

word retrieval, 79, 94
working memory subdomain, 2, 6, 35, 70, 95, 134, 151
    age effects, 80–81, *80*, 82–83, 103, 115
    brain function relations, 72–74, 106
    component of EF, 4, 6, 18, 29, 71–72
    components, 71
    convergent validity, 79, 80, 81–82, *81*, 137, *138*, 140
    data analysis, 80
    defined, 70–72
    discriminant validity, 79, 80, 81–82, *81*, 137, 139, *139*
    disruptions, 6, 72
    importance during childhood, 72
    method, 77–80
    participants, 77–78
    repeated testing, 81
    results, 80–82
    test/retest reliability, 81
    validation measure, 5, *13*, 19, 74–77, 78–79, 81–82, *81*, 83

CURRENT

National Institutes of Health Toolbox Cognition Battery (NIH Toolbox CB): Validation for Children Between 3 and 15 Years—*Philip David Zelazo and Patricia J. Bauer* (SERIAL NO. 309, 2013)

Resilience in Children With Incarcerated Parents—*Julie Poehlmann and J. Mark Eddy* (SERIAL NO. 308, 2013)

The Emergence of a Temporally Extended Self and Factors That Contribute to Its Development: From Theoretical and Empirical Perspectives—*Mary Lazaridis* (SERIAL NO. 307, 2013)

What Makes a Difference: Early Head Start Evaluation Findings in a Developmental Context—*John M. Love, Rachel Chazan-Cohen, Helen Raikes, and Jeanne Brooks-Gunn* (SERIAL NO. 306, 2013)

The Development of Mirror Self-Recognition in Different Sociocultural Contexts—*Joscha Kärtner, Heidi Keller, Nandita Chaudhary, and Relindis D. Yovsi* (SERIAL NO. 305, 2012)

"Emotions Are a Window Into One's Heart": A Qualitative Analysis of Parental Beliefs About Children's Emotions Across Three Ethnic Groups—*Alison E. Parker, Amy G. Halberstadt, Julie C. Dunsmore, Greg Townley, Alfred Bryant, Jr., Julie A. Thompson, and Karen S. Beale* (SERIAL NO. 304, 2012)

Physiological Measures of Emotion From a Developmental Perspective: State of the Science—*Tracy A. Dennis, Kristin A. Buss, and Paul D. Hastings* (SERIAL NO. 303, 2012)

How Socialization Happens on the Ground: Narrative Practices as Alternate Socializing Pathways in Taiwanese and European-American Families—*Peggy J. Miller, Heidi Fung, Shumin Lin, Eva Chian-Hui Chen, and Benjamin R. Boldt* (SERIAL NO. 302, 2012)

Children Without Permanent Parents: Research, Practice, and Policy—*Robert B. McCall, Marinus H. van IJzendoorn, Femmie Juffer, Christina J. Groark, and Victor K. Groza* (SERIAL NO. 301, 2011)

I Remember Me: Mnemonic Self-Reference Effects in Preschool Children—*Josephine Ross, James R. Anderson, and Robin N. Campbell* (SERIAL NO. 300, 2011)

Early Social Cognition in Three Cultural Contexts—*Tara Callaghan, Henrike Moll, Hannes Rakoczy, Felix Warneken, Ulf Liszkowski, Tanya Behne, and Michael Tomasello* (SERIAL NO. 299, 2011)

The Development of Ambiguous Figure Perception—*Marina C. Wimmer and Martin J. Doherty* (SERIAL NO. 298, 2011)

The Better Beinnings, Better Futures Project: Findings From Grade 3 to Grade 9—*Ray DeV. Peters, Alison J. Bradshaw, Kelly Petrunka, Geoffrey Nelson, Yves Herry, Wendy M. Craig, Robert Arnold, Kevin C. H. Parker, Shahriar R. Khan, Jeffrey S. Hoch, S. Mark Pancer, Colleen Loomis, Jean-Marc B´el anger , Susan Evers, Claire Maltais, Katherine Thompson, and Melissa D. Rossiter* (SERIAL NO. 297, 2010)

First-Year Maternal Employment and Child Development in the First 7 Years—*Jeanne Brooks- Gunn, Wen-Jui Han, and Jane Waldfogel* (SERIAL NO. 296, 2010)

Deprivation-Specific Psychological Patterns: Effects of Institutional Deprivation—*Michael Rutter, Edmund J. Sonuga-Barke, Celia Beckett, Jennifer Castle, Jana Kreppner, Robert Kumsta, Wolff Schlotz, Suzanne Stevens, and Christopher A. Bell* (SERIAL NO. 295, 2010)

A Dynamic Cascade Model of the Development of Substance-Use Onset—*Kenneth A. Dodge, Patrick S. Malone, Jennifer E. Lansford, Shari Miller, Gregory S. Pettit, and John E. Bates* (SERIAL NO. 294, 2009)

Flexibility in Early Verb Use: Evidence From a Multiple-N Diary Study—*Letitia R. Naigles, Erika Hoff, and Donna Vear* (SERIAL NO. 293, 2009)

Marital Conflict and Children's Externalizing Behavior: Interactions Between Parasympathetic and Sympathetic Nervous System Activity—*Mona El-Sheikh, Chrystyna D. Kouros, Stephen Erath, E. Mark Cummings, Peggy Keller, and Lori Staton* (SERIAL NO. 292, 2009)

The Effects of Early Social-Emotional and Relationship Experience on the Development of Young Orphanage Children—*The St. Petersburg–USA Orphanage Research Team* (SERIAL NO. 291, 2008)

Understanding Mother-Adolescent Conflict Discussions: Concurrent and Across-Time Prediction From Youths' Dispositions and Parenting—*Nancy Eisenberg, Claire Hofer, Tracy L. Spinrad, Elizabeth T. Gershoff, Carlos Valiente, Sandra Losoya, Qing Zhou, Amanda Cumberland, Jeffrey Liew, Mark Reiser, and Elizabeth Maxon* (SERIAL NO. 290, 2008)

Developing Object Concepts in Infancy: An Associative Learning Perspective—*David H. Rakison and Gary Lupyan* (SERIAL NO. 289, 2008)

The Genetic and Environmental Origins of Learning Abilities and Disabilities in the Early School Years—*Yulia Kovas, Claire M. A. Haworth, Philip S. Dale, and Robert Plomin* (SERIAL NO. 288, 2007)